Health Education
&
Community Pharmacy

Second Edition

Prof. N.K. Jain
M.Pharm., Ph.D., LL.M., F.I.C.

Director, I.S.F. College of Pharmacy,
Ferozepur G.T. Road, Moga - 142 001, Punjab
Formerly Professor & Head,
Department of Pharmaceutical Sciences,
Dr. H.S. Gour University, Sagar - 470 003, MP

CBS

CBS Publishers & Distributors Pvt Ltd

New Delhi • Bengaluru • Chennai • Kochi • Kolkata • Lucknow • Mumbai
Hyderabad • Jharkhand • Nagpur • Patna • Pune • Uttarakhand

Health Education and Community Pharmacy
Second Edition

ISBN: 978-81-239-2319-2

Copyright © Author and Publisher

Second Edition: 2015
Reprint: 2017, 2018, 2019, 2022, 2023
First Edition: 1996
Reprint: 2003, 2004, 2005, 2006, 2007, 2008, 2010

Published by Satish Kumar Jain and produced by Varun Jain for
CBS Publishers & Distributors Pvt Ltd
4819/XI Prahlad Street, 24 Ansari Road, Daryaganj, New Delhi 110 002, India
Ph: 011-23289259, 23266861   Website: www.cbspd.com
                                    e-mail: delhi@cbspd.com
Corporate Office: 204 FIE, Industrial Area, Patparganj, Delhi 110 092, India
Ph: 011-4934 4934   Fax: 011-4934 4935   e-mail: publishing@cbspd.com; publicity@cbspd.com

Branches

* **Bengaluru:** Seema House 2975, 17th Cross, KR Road, Banasankari 2nd Stage, Bengaluru 560 070, Karnataka, India
  Ph: +91-80-26771678/79   Fax: +91-80-26771680   e-mail: bangalore@cbspd.com
* **Chennai:** 7, Subbaraya Street, Shenoy Nagar, Chennai 600 030, Tamil Nadu, India
  Ph: +91-44-26680620, 26681266   Fax: +91-44-42032115   e-mail: chennai@cbspd.com
* **Kochi:** 42/1325, 1326, Power House Road, Opp KSEB, Power House, Ernakulam, Kochi 682 018, India
  Ph: +91-484-4059061–65   Fax: +91-484-4059065   e-mail: kochi@cbspd.com
* **Kolkata:** 147, Hind Ceramics Compound, 1st Floor, Nilgunj Road, Belghoria, Kolkata 700 056, West Bengal, India
  Ph: +91-33-25633055–56   e-mail: kolkata@cbspd.com
* **Lucknow:** Basement, Khushnuma Complex, 7-Meerabai Marg (behind Jawahar Bhawan), Lucknow 226 001, India
  Ph: +91-522-4000032   e-mail: tiwari.lucknow@cbspd.com
* **Mumbai:** PWD Shed. Gala no. 25/26, Ramchandra Bhatt Marg, Next to JJ Hospital Gate no. 2, Opp. Union Bank of India, Noorbaug Mumbai 400 009, Maharashtra, India
  Ph: +91-22-66661880/89   e-mail: mumbai@cbspd.com

Representatives

* **Hyderabad** 0-9885175004 • **Jharkhand** 0-9811541605   • **Nagpur**   0-9421945513
* **Patna**   0-9334159340 • **Pune**   0-9923910676   • **Uttarakhand** 0-9716462459

Printed at Glorious Printers, Jhilmil Industrial Area, Delhi, India

Preface to the Second Edition

Health education and community pharmacy are undergoing transformation in view of growing public awareness as well as recent advances. The role of a pharmacist is also being much more appreciated and emphasized in terms of newer drugs and delivery systems as well as recognition of the health care needs of the growing population.

Consumer Protection Act and Right to Information Act have increased the accountability of all members of health care team, including pharmacists.

The first edition of this book was published in 1996 and since then it has been reprinted eight times. This establishes the popularity of the book and hence an attempt has been made to update the information.

The second edition has undergone highly significant changes in terms of the subject matter, treatment of the topics and formatting, so as to make it more useful to students and teachers. Description of few diseases has been added to keep pace with the time. Liberal addition of figures will facilitate the learning objective. Glossary is a new addition that will serve as a handy compilation of definitions of common terms. The question bank has been greatly expanded.

It is expected that this thoroughly revised edition will provide up-to-date knowledge and meet the requirements of both Diploma and Degree students.

I would like to acknowledge my students Miss Keerti Jain and Mr Vijay Mishra for their assistance, and M/s CBS Publishers and Distributors for meticulous printing of this book.

Suggestions and criticisms from any corner shall be appreciated and duly acknowledged.

Sagar, 07 Jan, 2015   Professor N.K. Jain

Contents

Solid Waste Disposal and Control, Disposal of Sewage, Medical
Entomology, Arthropod-Borne Diseases and Their Control,
Rodents, Animals and Diseases.

Concepts of Health and Disease

INTRODUCTION

'Health is wealth' is taught to us since childhood. Thus health is of concern to every individual, community, state and nation and now it has attained global status. But the concept of health varies widely. Pharmacist as an individual as well as a member of health care team is much more actively concerned with the concept of health. In 1977 the World Health Assembly resolved that the main social target of governments and WHO (World Health Organization) in the coming decades should be 'the attainment by all citizens of the world by the year 2000 of a level of health that will permit them to lead a socially and economically productive life'. Thus "Health for all by 2000 AD' was adopted as internationally attainable target. It was not merely a slogan but recognition of the importance of health in national and international perspective. Unfortunately India failed in attaining this objective. In 1979 the United Nations adopted health as an integral part of socio-economic development.

Health has evolved as a concept over centuries from an individual concern to a global social goal. The concept of health is dynamic. As all other concepts change and the newer concepts emerge, the concept of health also keeps on changing. The members of a community including professional groups like health administrators, scientists, ecologists, politicians, etc perceive it in different ways. This obviously leads to confusion and we come across different concepts of health. These concepts include the definitions of a health norm and a systematic way of identifying and dealing with the deviations. **Disease** is considered as a deviation from normal.

CONCEPTS OF HEALTH

Important concepts of health are discussed below:

A. Biomedical Concept

This concept is based on the **germ theory of disease**. The medical profession perceives the human body as a machine, disease as a consequence of the breakdown of the machine, and one of the doctor's tasks being to repair the machine. However the biomedical concept is found inadequate to solve major health problems like accidents, chronic diseases, malnutrition, mental illness, population explosion, drug abuse, environmental pollution etc.

B. Ecological Concept

The ecologists consider health as a dynamic equilibrium between man and the environment and disease as maladjustment of the human organism to environment. According to Dubos 'health implies the relative absence of pain and discomfort and a continuous adaptation and adjustment to ensure optimal function'. We must appreciate that human ecological and cultural adaptations do determine the occurrence of diseases as well as the availability of food and population explosion. It is believed that greater human adaptation to natural environments can result in longer life expectancies and a better quality of life even in the absence of modern health delivery systems. Recently there has been an increasing recognition for 'environmental friendly' products including pharmaceutical and specially packaging materials.

C. Psychological Concept

According to this concept health is both a biological as well as social phenomenon because it is influenced by social, psychological, cultural, economical, and political factors. Psychological and social considerations are important in concept of health.

D. Holistic Concept

It represents the synthesis of all the above concepts. It takes into account all the factors influencing the health such as social, economic, political and environmental. This concept is descried as a unified and multidimensional process involving the well being of the whole person in the context of his environment. It implies that all sectors of society have an influence on health e.g. agriculture, animal husbandry, food, industry, education, housing, public works, communication etc. The holistic concept is mainly concerned with the promotion and protection of public health.

The preference for different theories varies by such social and demographic characteristics as education, occupation, income and ethnic group membership. As drug experts, pharmacists can play an important role in clarifying to the patients the points on which folk or coexistent therapies may be in conflict with scientific procedure.

DEFINITION OF HEALTH

Health has been defined in various ways and hence there exist a number of definitions. However a perfect definition is still not settled mainly because different people view it in different perspectives.

According to WHO 'health is a state of complete physical, mental and social well being and not merely an absence of disease or infirmity'. But this definition is criticized as being idealistic but not practical because according to this definition all of us are sick and no body is healthy!

According to Oxford English dictionary health is 'soundness of body or mind, that condition in which its functions are duly and effectively discharged'.

According to Webster dictionary 'health is the condition of being sound in body, mind or spirit, especially freedom from physical disease and pain'.

According to the modern philosophy 'health is a fundamental right and it is the essence of productive life. It involves individual, national and international responsibility.

MODELS FOR HEALTH DESCRIPTION

A model is a theoretical way of understanding a concept or idea. It represents different ways of approaching complex issues. Health beliefs are a person's ideas, convictions, and attitudes about health and illness. Because health beliefs usually influence health behaviour, they can affect a client's health positively or negatively. 'Prevention of illness' is a positive health behaviour. Common positive health behaviours include immunization, proper sleep patterns, adequate exercise, and nutrition. Preventing illness is one aspect of wellness care that focuses on detection or prevention of disease. Different models used to describe health are as follow:

A. Clinical Model

- The absence of signs and symptoms of disease indicates health.
- Illness would be the presence of conspicuous signs and symptoms of disease.

People who use this model of health to guide their use of healthcare services may not seek preventive health services, or they may wait until they are very ill to seek care.

B. Role Performance Model

- Health is indicated by the ability to perform social roles.
- Role performance includes work, family and social roles, with performance based on society expectations.
- Illness would be the failure to perform a person's roles at the level of others in society.
- This model is basis for work and physical examination by a physician.
- The sick role, in which people can be excused from performing their social roles while they are ill, is a vital component of the role performance model.

C. Adaptive Model

- The ability to adapt positively to social, mental, and physiological changes is indicative of health.
- Illness occurs when the person fails to adapt or becomes unadaptive toward these changes.

D. Agent-Host-Environmental Model

- This model was postulated by Leavell and Clark in 1965.
- It is useful for examining causes of disease in an individual.
- The agent, host and environment interact in ways that create risk factors, and understanding these is important for the promotion and maintenance of health.
- An agent is an environmental factor or stressor that must be present or absent for an illness to occur.
- A host is a living organism capable of being infected or affected by an agent.
- The host reaction is influenced by family history, age, and health habits.

E. High Level Wellness Model

- It was proposed by Dunn in 1961.
- It recognizes health as an ongoing process toward a person's highest potential of functioning. This process involves the person, family and the community.
- It describes high-level wellness as "the experience of a person alive with the glow of good health, alive to the tips of their fingers with energy to burn, tingling with vitality – at times like this the world is a glorious place".

F. Holistic Health Model

- It was proposed by Edelman and Mandle in 2002.
- Holism acknowledges and respects the interaction of a person's mind, body and spirit within the environment. Holism is an antidote to the atomistic approach of contemporary science. An atomistic approach takes things apart, examining the person piece by piece in an attempt to understand the larger picture.
- Holism is based on the belief that people (or their parts) can not be fully understood if examined solely in pieces apart from their environment.

G. Nightingale's Theory of Environment

- It was postulated by Florence Nightingale.
- This model views health as a constantly changing state, with high level wellness and death being on opposite ends of a graduated scale, or continuum.
- This continuum illustrates the dynamic state of health, as a person adapts to changes in the internal and external environments to maintain a state of well-being. A patient with chronic illness may view himself/herself at different points of the continuum at any given time, depending on how well the patient believes he/she is functioning with.

DIMENSIONS OF HEALTH

Health is **multidimensional**, important dimensions being physical, mental, social and spiritual. Other dimensions could be emotional, vocational, political etc. Each dimension functions and interacts with each other but has certain characteristics.

A. Physical Health

Physical health is easier to understand. It represents a biological state of fitness in which every cell and every organ of the body is functioning at optimum capacity and in perfect harmony with the rest of the body. Thus physical health implies absence of an evident disease.

It is characterized by normal functioning of the body organs e.g. normal blood pressure, normal liver functioning, normal skin and so on. A **nomogram** correlating the average height with average weight could be used as an indicator of physical health. It should be remembered that physical health is assessed in terms of age and sex of an individual by comparing, for example, the vital capacity of his lung with the reported normal value for that age and sex.

B. Mental Health

Mental health has been defined as a state of balance between the individual and the surrounding world, a state of harmony between oneself and others, a coexistence between the realities of self and that of other people, and that of environment. Mental health is difficult to assess. It is certainly not mere absence of disease and is influenced by psychological factors. Schizophrenia and depression are examples of mental illness. Mental illness can also lead to physical illness, for example, mental tension may lead to peptic ulcer. Similarly physical illness can also lead to mental illness, for example, a leprotic person may suffer from depression. Exact assessment of mental health is difficult but approximate comparisons are possible by assessing the mental functioning. Positive mental health is one of the keys to good health.

C. Social Health

Social health is defined as the quantity and quality of an individual's interpersonal ties and the extent of involvement with the community. It recognizes the fact that every individual is part of the society and takes into consideration the social and economic conditions and well being of the 'whole person' in the context of his social network. Social health involves harmony and integration with the individual, between each individual and other members of society and between individuals and the world in which he lives.

D. Spiritual Health

It is a relatively newer concept and hence not properly defined. Spiritual dimension of health includes integrity, principles and ethics, purpose in life, commitment to some higher being and belief in concepts that are not subject to the 'state-of-art' explanation. It refers to that part of the individual, which reaches out and strives for meaning and purpose in life. It is related to the 'spirit', the sole. All religions and religious leaders consider the attainment of spiritual health as the ultimate goal of life.

In addition to the above, health could also be defined in terms of many other dimensions such as nutritional, socio-economic, environmental, emotional, vocational etc. The WHO definition of health as 'a state of complete physical, mental and social well-being and not merely an absence of disease' is broad and covers most of the dimensions of health, directly or indirectly.

DETERMINANTS OF HEALTH

Health of an individual is not static; it is a dynamic phenomenon and a process of continuous change. It is a state, which is to be attained first and then maintained. Health fluctuates within a range of optimum well being to various levels of deficiencies including death. Disease may manifest itself at any time of life.

Factors which either alone or in combination are responsible for diseases include genetics, infective organisms, nutritional deficiencies, metabolic disturbances, allergic disorders, aging and degenerative processes, cancer and other neoplasm, iatrogenesis, accidental injuries and social pathology. The health of individuals and communities may be considered as the result of interactions due to genetic and environmental factors.

More important determinants of health are given below:

A. Heredity

Besides other factors, health is also dependent on the genetic make up of an individual. These inborn factors play a part in determining life-span and likelihood of developing certain illnesses. In this context health is defined as 'that state of the individual, which is based upon the absence from the genetic constitution of genes that cause serious defect or the presence in the genetic constitution of the genes, which correspond to the normal characterization". It is the nature of genes at the time of conception, which governs the characteristics of an individual. This is the reason why most of the genetic diseases are difficult to cure. Common diseases of genetic origin are mental retardation, errors of metabolism and chromosomal anomalies. Scientists all over the world are attempting to synthesize genes, which are best in every respect including health as genetic heritage.

B. Environment

A pharmacist knows very well that environment has a direct impact on the physical, mental and social well being of those living in it. The physical environment constitutes a varying range of natural factors like climate, soils, forests, rivers, rainfall etc. The people and their actions as indicated by traditions, customs and superstitions represent the social aspect of environment. Biological environment comprises plants and animals including bacteria, viruses, parasites and pathogens, which cause disease. Full use of one's physical and mental capabilities can be realized only in a favorable environment. All countries of the world are seriously concerned with the promotion and protection of family and environmental health. Clean environment is absolutely essential for good health.

The internal environment is concerned with each and every component part, every tissue, every organ, and organ system and their harmonious functioning within the system.

The **external environment** or **macroenvironment** is defined as 'all that which is external to the individual host' and consists of those things to which man is exposed after conception.

Personal environment pertaining to individual's way of living and life style e.g. eating habits, smoking or drinking, exercise etc; is sometimes called **microenvironment** or **domestic environment**.

C. Life Style

Life style is composed of cultural and behavioural patterns and life-long habits. It plays an important role in the presentation of health. Thus health can be viewed as the quality of life that enables the individual to live most and serve best. Habit is called second nature. Habits are largely responsible for determining one's life style. Life styles are learnt through social interaction, school and mass media. Healthy life styles would include adequate nutrition, sufficient sleep, enough physical activity etc. Smoking, alcoholism and 'drugs' constitute negative life style, not conducive to health.

D. Socio-Economic Conditions

Socio-economic conditions like per capita GNP (Gross National Product), education, economic status, political system, employment, housing etc have a great deal of influence on the human health. These factors are multiple, interactive and very often go beyond the extent of individual's control. Integrated and multi-levels of public health interventions are crucial to shape these factors for a positive health impact. Educated people better appreciate the importance of health. Health status improves with level of education. Education is closely tied to socio-economic status. It increases opportunities for job and income security, improves people's ability to access and understand information to help them keep healthy. Education improves the overall human attitude to health. Low mortality rate in Kerala is partly due to high literacy rate. The economic status as indicated by per capita GNP also influences the health status. Higher income and status generally results in greater control and discretion. Income determines living conditions such as safe housing and ability to buy sufficient good food thus better economic status can be responsible for reduced mortality rate, increased life expectancy and improved quality of life. WHO has set up the target of at least 5% expenditure out of GNP of a country on health care. This is possible only if the political system in the country is committed to provide improved health care by framing and implementing prior policies and by allocating necessary funds. Unless the political leaders make serious efforts, the health development would be difficult. It is equally important to realize that factors like housing, sanitation, nutrition, employment etc also contribute in the overall socio-economic conditions.

E. Health and Family Welfare Services

Health services must improve health care and health. The extent to which health services are provided is directly reflected in terms of life expectancy and various mortality rates. Health services should be available at reasonable cost and equally to all individuals starting from pregnant women, infants, adults, males and females, cancer patients, mentally retarded people etc. In India the Ministry of Health and Family Welfare is responsible for planning and implementing health services. Primary Health Centers (PHCs) at village level, family welfare schemes, hospitals etc all help in improving health services. Health services must be effective.

F. Other Factors

Health is a resultant of so many factors including the primary factors discussed above. In addition, there are other factors outside the formal health care system such as rural development, social welfare, food and agriculture, industry, economic and social policies, which should assist in improving the standard of living and ultimately the health status of individuals, the society, the nation and the world. Pharmacist is a part of health care team as one who is an expert on drugs and related matters.

As people's health is influenced by a wide range of factors, which go beyond the health care sector; therefore, community participation and inter-sectoral cooperation are required to integrate health promotion actions and transform health determinants for the better. The healthy cities project provides an excellent platform to enable concerted effort of all sectors of the community to work together in partnership to improve health in the place where we live, work and love.

INDICATORS OF HEALTH

Indicators of health are used to assess the health status of a distinct population, for example a community, district, state, country; and compare it with other community, district, state or country. According to WHO 'indicators are variables, which help to measure changes'. Indicators are expressed as rates for a particular base over a definite period of time. The general formula for a rate of any type is:

$$\text{Rate} = \frac{\text{No. of events measured}}{\text{Population at risk}} \times K$$

where K is a constant and multiple of time.

Such indicators are helpful in monitoring and evaluation of health services, activities and programmes. Such indicators of health can assess the success or failure of any health programme.

A. Groups of Health Indicators

Ideal indicators of health should be *valid, reliable, sensitive* and *specific*. Main groups of health indicators are discussed below:

(a) Morbidity indicators

Morbidity means any departure from a state of well being due to a disease, an injury or any impairment. Morbidity indicators are used to supplement mortality data to describe the health status of a population. Morbidity indicators in common use are explained below:

(i) Incidence Rate

Rate of incidence of any disease either for the number of persons or spells of sickness can be calculated as:

$$\text{Incidence Rate} = \frac{\text{No. of cases of sickness starting during the period in an area}}{\text{Average No. of persons exposed to risk during that period in that area}} \times 1000$$

(ii) Prevalence Rate

It measures the extent of total prevalence of a disease during a period (whether starting before or during that period). **Point Prevalence Rate** gives the rate at a point of time whereas **Period Prevalence Rate** gives the rate for a period of time. It is calculated as:

$$\text{Period Prevalence Rate} = \frac{\text{No. of cases of a disease prevalent at any time (or period) in the area}}{\text{Average No. of persons exposed to the risk during that point (or period) of time}} \times 1000$$

(iii) Case Fatality Rate

It measures the extent of fatality of any disease, for example, the proportion of deaths from disease to the reported cases of that disease.

$$\text{Case Fatality Rate} = \frac{\text{No. of people who die of a disease}}{\text{No. of people who have the disease}}$$

(b) Mortality Indicators

Mortality represents expectancy of life at various ages etc. Obviously it takes into consideration the number of deaths out of a definite population. Mortality indicators represent the traditional measures of health status. The rate can be calculated for any age or sex group or both, in an area, during a year. Common mortality indicators are calculated as follows.

(i) $\qquad$ Crude Death Rate $= \dfrac{\text{No. of deaths during the year}}{\text{Mid year population}} \times 1000$

(ii) $\qquad$ Age and Sex-Specific Death Rate $= \dfrac{\begin{array}{c}\text{No. of deaths registered or estimated in an}\\ \text{age and sex group during a year in an area}\end{array}}{\begin{array}{c}\text{Estimated population of that age and sex}\\ \text{group for the year in that area}\end{array}} \times 1000$

(iii) $\qquad$ Infant Mortality Rate $= \dfrac{\begin{array}{c}\text{No. of deaths registered or estimated of children}\\ \text{below one year of age during a year in area}\end{array}}{\begin{array}{c}\text{No. of live births registered or estimated}\\ \text{during the year in the area}\end{array}} \times 1000$

Similarly neo-natal and pre-natal mortality rates can also be calculated.

(c) Sullivan's Index

It is the most advanced indicator based on the expectation of life, free of disability. It is calculated as:

Sullivan's Index = Life expectancy (years) – Duration of bed disability and inability (years) to perform major activities

Thus if the life expectancy is 60 years and bed disability and inability to perform major activities is 5 years then Sullivan's index would be 60 – 5 = 55 years.

CONCEPT OF DISEASE

Disease is just opposite to health. The word could be dissected as *dis* and *ease* meaning opposite to ease, or uneasiness. Disease can be defined as 'an impairment of the normal state of the living being that affects the performance of the vital functions'. It is also defined as 'a pathological condition of the body that presents a group of symptoms peculiar to it and which sets the condition apart as an abnormal entity differing from other normal or pathological body states'.

Like health, disease is also viewed differently by different people or groups. From a sociological point of view disease is considered a social phenomenon occurring in all societies.

From an ecological point of view disease is maladjustment of the human organism to the environment.

The terms disease, illness and sickness have been used synonymously but they are actually different. Whereas **disease** is a physiological/psychological dysfunction, **illness** is a subjective state of the person who feels aware of not being well; and sickness is a state of social dysfunction, a role that an individual assumes when ill (sickness role).

Diseases could be physical, mental (psychological) or social. They could be caused by bacteria and viruses, insects and animal bites, strain, accident, injury etc.

Surprisingly WHO has not defined the term disease!

NATURAL HISTORY OF DISEASE

Natural history of disease refers to the progress of a disease process in an individual over time, in the absence of intervention. The process begins with exposure to or accumulation of factors capable of causing disease. Without medical intervention, the process ends with recovery, disability, or death (Fig. 1.1).

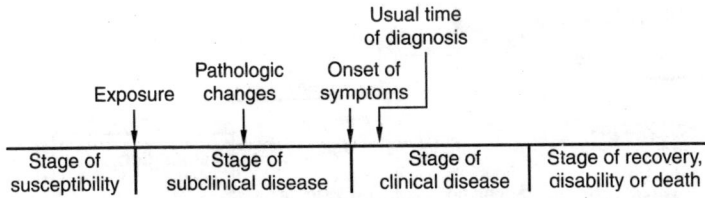

Fig. 1.1. Different stages of a disease.

Natural history of a disease traces the sequence of event in the evolution of a disease; from the initial stage of its pre-pathogenesis phase to its termination as recovery, disability or death in the absence of treatment or prevention. The natural history of one disease differs from another. Similarly, the natural history of a disease may also differ in individuals. It is a key concept in epidemiology.

Natural history of a disease comprises of two phases, (a) pre-pathogenesis (progress in the environment), and (b) pathogenesis (progress in the human beings). Thus natural history of a disease gives us an idea as to how and why a disease is caused and how can it be prevented or cured.

A. Pre-pathogenesis Phase

Every disease is an interaction between **man**, the **causative agent** of the disease and the **environment**. Pre-pathogenesis phase signifies the period when the disease agent has not actually entered man but the factors favourable to its interaction with human host already exist in the environment. Thus the situation could be described as 'man exposed to the risk of disease'. In this way all of us are in the pre-pathogenesis phase of most of the communicable and non-communicable diseases!

B. Pathogenesis Phase

In this phase the disease agent actually enters the susceptible human host and in case of infectious diseases it multiplies and induces tissue and physiological changes. Recovery, disability or death of the host may follow this. Immunization and chemotherapy serve as intervening measures in pathogenesis phase. The infection may be clinical or sub-clinical or the host may become a **carrier** with or without developing clinical disease, for example, poliomyelitis and diphtheria. In chronic diseases such as cancer, hypertension, coronary heart diseases this phase normally consists of a pre-symptomatic phase and a symptomatic phase. In the **pre-symptomatic phase** there are no recognizable symptoms and there is no manifest disease but in the **symptomatic phase** the disease has already well advanced. A sequence of events in the natural history of a disease is shown in detail in Fig. 1.2 and the iceberg of disease is shown in Fig. 1.3.

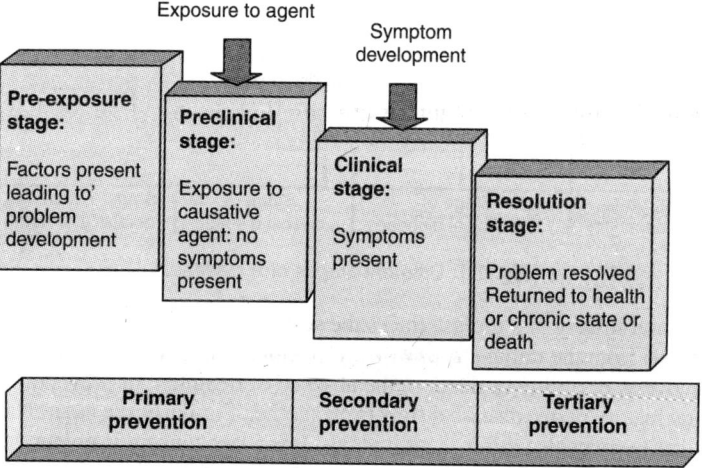

Fig. 1.2. Natural history of a disease.

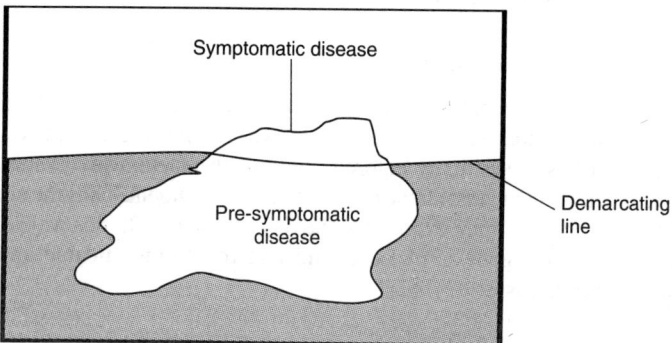

Fig. 1.3. Iceberg of disease.

According to the concept of iceberg of disease, disease in a community may be compared with an iceberg. The floating tip of the iceberg represents what the physician sees in the community. The tip represents those persons who have shown symptoms of the disease and are recognized as cases (diseased persons). The vast submerged portion of the iceberg represents the hidden mass of the disease that is latent/inapparent/pre-symptomatic/undiagnosed cases and carriers in the community. The water line represents the demarcation between clinical and subclinical or undiagnosed patients.

In some cases (for example, hypertension, diabetes, anemia, malnutrition and mental illness) the unknown morbidity (represented by submerged portion of iceberg) far exceeds the known morbidity. Thus detection and control of undiagnosed reservoir of disease is a challenge to modern technique.

The disease agent: The word etiology is derived from words *aitia* meaning cause and *ology* meaning science. Hence etiology is the scientific study of the causes of disease. Disease agent is the first link in the chain of disease transmission. It is the most important factor causing the disease (Fig. 1.4).

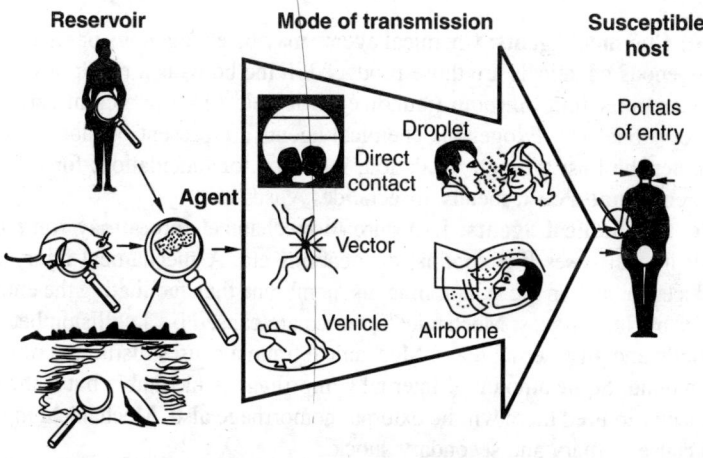

Fig. 1.4. Chain of infection.

The disease agent is defined as "a living or non-living substance or a tangible or intangible force, the excessive prevalence or selective lacks of which may initiate or perpetuate a disease process". A disease may have a single agent, a number of independent alternative agents or a complex of two or more factors whose combined presence is essential for the development of a disease.

C. Classification of Etiological Factors

(a) Biological agents: Viruses, rickettsiae, fungi, bacteria etc are the biological agents of disease. These agents exhibit (a) **infectivity** (the ability of an infectious agent to invade, multiply and produce infection in a host), (b)

pathogenicity (the ability to induce clinically apparent illness), and (c) **virulence** (the degree of pathogenicity). Such agents can multiply in the body and exaggerate the initial danger. They can spread the disease in different parts of the body and produce toxins.

(b) **Nutrient agents:** Any excess or deficiency of nutrient agent may result in nutritional disorders. Examples of nutrient agents include carbohydrates, fats, proteins, vitamins, minerals, enzymes and water; and examples of nutritional problems are anemia, goiter, obesity, night blindness, protein energy malnutrition etc. Dietary deficiency may lower body resistance against infectious diseases.

(c) **Physical agents:** Physical agents like heat, cold, humidity, radiation, electricity, sound etc may also cause illness. Severe cold can depress the functional efficacy of the ciliated epithelium of the respiratory tract, allowing the passage of bacteria into the lungs. Exposure of whole body to severe heat in combination with humidity can result into a heat stroke. Over exposure to ultraviolet rays causes burns. High voltage currents may cause instantaneous death.

(d) **Chemical agents:** Chemical agents may be endogenous or exogenous. Endogenous chemicals are those produced in the body as a result of disease, for example serum bilirubin (jaundice), uric acid (gout), calcium carbonate (kidney stone) etc. Exogenous chemical agents are present outside the body but enter the host through inhalation, ingestion, or inoculation; for example allergens, fumes, dust, metals, insecticides, gases etc.

(e) **Mechanical agents:** Exposure to mechanical forces may sometimes result into diseases like sprains, dislocations etc. A mechanical injury may produce a breach in the skin or mucous membrane thus facilitating the entry of organisms into tissues. Mechanical injuries are caused by a collision between the body and an external mass. Mechanical trauma causes disruption of tissue or a wound. Some amount of internal hemorrhage is inevitable but if the skin has been ruptured there will be external hemorrhage also. Mechanical injuries also cause primary and secondary shock.

(f) **Social agents:** These are the social factors, which play a role in the occurrence of disease. Unhygienic living conditions, unhealthy life styles, poverty, illiteracy and lack of awareness, smoking, abuse of drugs and alcohol etc are the examples of social agents.

CONCEPT OF PREVENTION OF DISEASE

Prevention is always better than cure. A proper understanding of the natural history of disease and the agents, which cause them, will be useful in adopting preventive measures against diseases. The object of preventive medicine is to intercept the 'cause' and hence the disease processes. Prevention could be better understood by dividing it into (A) primary prevention, (B) secondary prevention, and (C) tertiary prevention.

A. Primary Prevention

It includes the concept of positive health and signifies intervention in the pre-pathogenesis phase of a disease. It is defined as action taken before the onset of disease, which rules out the possibility that a disease will ever occur. Primary prevention is based on measures, which promote general health, quality of life of people, or by protective measures such as literacy campaigns, education, and food production. For the primary prevention of chronic diseases WHO has recommended the following approaches if the 'risk factors' are established. The term 'risk factor' is used to describe the etiology of a disease when the disease agent is not clearly established. It is defined as 'an activity or exposure that is significantly associated with the development of a disease'. It is also defined as a determinant that can be modified by intervention, thereby reducing the possibility of occurrence of disease or other specified outcome.

(a) **Primordial prevention:** Primordial prevention is of special interest in prevention of chronic diseases. It is the primary prevention in the real sense. In this approach efforts are directed towards discouraging children from adopting harmful life styles mainly through individual and mass education. For example, the diseases like hypertension and obesity have their origin in early childhood when the life styles are formed e.g. eating habits, unhygienic habits, physical exercise, smoking etc.

(b) **Population (mass) strategy:** The population strategy is directed towards the life styles, socio-economic and behavioral changes in the whole population irrespective of individual risk levels. Thus it has been proved that even a small reduction in the average blood pressure of a population would produce a large reduction in the incidence of cardiovascular diseases. Similarly an increase in the average income of a population suffering from malnutrition would improve the health status of the population.

(c) **High-risk strategy:** In any population there may be certain individuals who may be at high risk. High-risk strategy is based on the detection of individuals at high-risk by optimum use of clinical methods. AIDS is a relatively new fatal disease but its rate of spread is alarming. Better control of this disease would anticipate detection of individuals at high-risk and taking preventive care in such cases.

B. Secondary Prevention

Secondary prevention is related to the preventive measures taken *after* the occurrence of disease to arrest the disease process and restore health. It can also help in protecting the individuals who have not acquired the disease so far. Hence secondary prevention can prevent spread of infection in already infected persons and at the same time potential contacts get primary prevention. Secondary prevention can be defined as 'action that halts the progress of a disease at its incipient stage and prevents complications'. These actions include early diagnosis, adequate treatment, Governmental Health programmes etc.

However secondary prevention is an imperfect tool. It is more expensive and less effective than primary prevention. The patient has already suffered from mental anguish, physical pain and the community has been subjected to loss of productivity. This does not happen in primary prevention. Thus long-term health policy would lay greater emphasis on primary prevention as compared to secondary prevention. Primary prevention is safer and least costly.

C. Tertiary Prevention

It is defined as 'all measures available to reduce or limit impairments and disabilities, minimizing suffering caused by existing departures from good health and to promote the patient's adjustment to intermediate condition'. Tertiary prevention means intervention in the late pathogenesis stage as when the disease process has crossed its early stages. Tertiary prevention, if undertaken in the natural history of disease, may prevent sequel and limit disability. This can be followed by rehabilitation programmes. Tertiary prevention extends the concept of prevention into fields of rehabilitation. Modern day rehabilitation programmes include psychological, vocational and medical components involving the team wok of a variety of professionals.

As per the natural history of disease, epidemiology has derived 3 levels of prevention of disease, which are summarized in Table 1.1.

Table 1.1. Levels of prevention of disease

Primary Prevention	Secondary Prevention	Tertiary Prevention
(a) Health Promotion: Through health education, nutritional intervention, life style, behavioural changes and regular exercises. **(b) Specific Protection:** Through immunization, chemoprophylaxis, nutritional supplements, pollution free environment, noise control, standardization of consumer products and accident control.	**(a) Early Diagnosis:** Regular checkup of community. **(b) Prompt treatment:** Proper treatment of diagnosed diseases. **(c) Prevent complications.**	**(a) Disability Limitation:** Through proper exercise, physio- and occupational therapy, corrective plastic surgery to improve mobility. **(b) Rehabilitation:** Mental and physical makeup to become productive, establishing independence and status in the society.

HEALTH CARE IN INDIA – VISION 2020

Good health confers on a person or groups freedom from illness - and the ability to realize one's potential. Health is therefore best understood as the indispensable basis for defining a person's sense of well being.

Health care covers not merely medical care but also all aspects of preventive care. It can not be limited to care rendered by or financed out of public expenditure within the government sector alone but must include incentives and disincentives for self care and care paid for by private citizens to get over ill health.

Health care system should include the following criteria for making it ideal;. first, universal access, and access to an adequate level without excessive burden; second, fair distribution of financial costs for access and fair distribution of burden in rationing care and capacity and a constant search for improvement to a more than just a system; third, training providers for competence empathy and accountability, pursuit of quality care and cost effective use of the results of relevant research; and lastly, special attention to vulnerable groups such as children, women, disabled and the aged.

In this context we may refer to the large ratio-based rural health infrastructure consisting of over 5 lakh trained doctors working under rural systems of medicine and a vast frontline force of over 7 lakh Auxiliary Nurse Midwife (ANMs), Multipurpose workers (MPWS) and *Anganwadi* workers besides community volunteers. The creation of such public work force should be seen as a major achievement in a country short of resources and struggling with great disparities in health status. As part of rural primary health care network alone, a total of 1.6 lakh subcenters, (with 1.27 lakh ANMs in position) and 22975 Primary Health Centres (PHCs) and 2935 Community Health Centres (CHCs) (with over 24000 doctors and over 3500 specialists to serve in them) have been set up. To promote Indian systems of medicine and homeopathy, there are over 22000 dispensaries, 2800 hospitals besides 6 lakh *Angawadis* serve nutrition needs of nearly 20 million children and 4 million mothers. The total effort has cost the bulk of the health development outlay, which stood at over Rs 62.5 crores or 3.64% of total plan spending during the last fifty years.

We have already the distinction of elimination or control acceptable to public health standards of small pox and guinea worm diseases. In the draft of National Health Policy-2001 it was proposed to eliminate or control the following diseases within limits acceptable to public health practice.

- Polio and leprosy by 2005.
- Kala-azar and Filariasis by 2010, which seems feasible due to its localized prevalence and the possibility of greater community based work.
- Blindness prevalence to 0.5% by 2010 seems less feasible due to a growing population. At present the programme is massively supported by foreign aid as there are many other legitimate demands on domestic health budgets.
- AIDS reaching zero growth by 2007 appears to be problematic as there are disputes even about base data on infected population. On most reckonings, affordable vaccines are not likely to be available soon nor do anti-retroviral drugs appear likely at affordable prices in the near future. Further the prevalence curve of AIDS in India is yet to show its shape.

Apart from the above, there remains a vast unfinished burden in preventing, controlling or eliminating other major communicable diseases and in bringing down the risk of deaths in maternal and peri-natal conditions. Endemic diseases arising from infection or lack of nutrition continue to account for almost two thirds of mortality and morbidity in India.

For achieving the goal of Good health for all, current PHC (Primary) and CHC (Community Health Centres) budgets may have to be increased by 10% per year for five years to draw level. A National Health Policy was first formulated in 1983 and an updated Health Policy was introduced in 2002. The main objective of the Policy is to achieve an acceptable standard of good health amongst the general population by the country. The National Health Policy 2002 sets out an allocation of 55% of the total public health investment for the primary health sector, 35% for secondary health sector and 10% for tertiary health sector. The policy has also planned health sector expenditure to 6% of GDP (Gross Domestic Product).

A pharmacist having adequate knowledge of these concepts of health and disease would be more useful to the country.

Nutrition and Health

INTRODUCTION

In the previous chapter we learnt that 'health is not merely an absence of disease' and that it is 'a condition of being sound in body, mind or spirit'. The level of general public health in India is not satisfactory but it has been improving over the years. Food and nutrition are important in maintaining good health.

A **food** may be defined as 'any substance which when taken into the body, can be utilized to yield heat or energy, to build up new tissues and to repair worn-out tissues, to regulate body processes and to aid in the production of important body compounds'.

Nutrition may be defined as 'the science of food and its relationship to health'. It is concerned primarily with the part played by nutrients in body growth, development and maintenance.

In attaining the target 'health for all', promotion of proper health is an important element of primary health care. Today we are better informed about the association of nutrition with infection, immunity, fertility, maternal and child health and family health. Nutritional indicators have been developed to monitor health for all.

CLASSIFICATION OF FOODS

Foods can be classified in many ways as shown in Fig. 2.1.

NUTRITIONAL LEVELS

Adequate nutrition enables individuals to grow, mature, reproduce and function in a healthy and normal manner. **Under nutrition** is a shortage in the total essential nutrients in the diet caused by an insufficient supply of food.

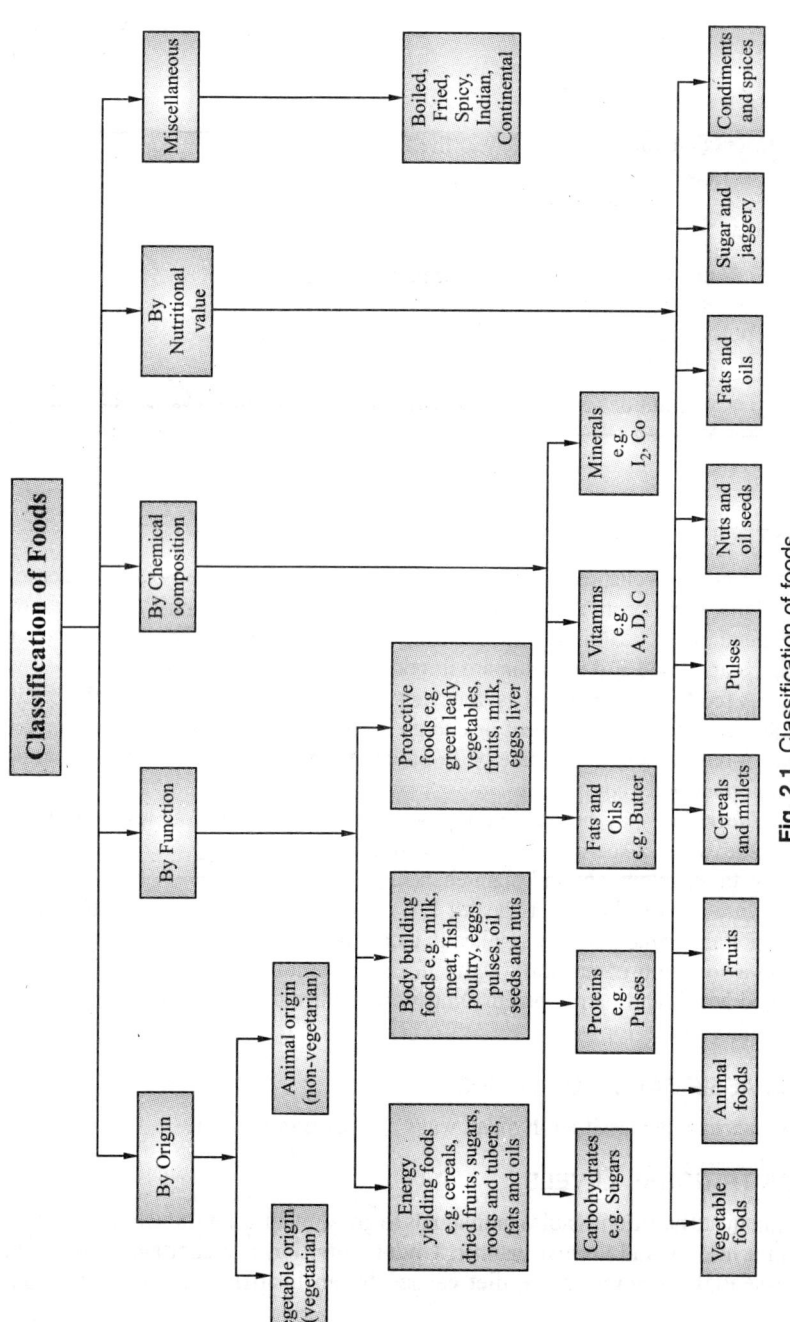

Fig. 2.1. Classification of foods.

Malnutrition means bad nutrition whether due to deficiency or excess of one or more nutrients.

NUTRITIONAL REQUIREMENTS

An adequate diet should perform the following functions:

1. It must supply energy for the basal metabolism as well as muscular and other work of the body.
2. It must supply energy and material for the synthesis of structural components necessary for optimum growth.
3. It must supply agents necessary to perform chemical reactions in the above processes.
4. It must supply energy and chemicals for reproduction.

The amount of nutrients needed for the body can be expressed in terms of **Recommended Daily Allowance** (RDA) or **Recommended Daily Intake** (RDI). RDA is defined as 'the amounts of nutrients sufficient for the maintenance of health in nearly all people'. *RDA of different nutrients vary according to the age, sex and special conditions like pregnancy and lactating mothers.*

Common nutritional requirements include proteins, vitamins and minerals.

PROTEINS

Proteins are most essential for the maintenance of human life. Tissues, muscles, organs, enzymes and hormones are protein in nature. The body can't store excess protein. Protein requirement is expressed in terms of grams/kg body weight. The daily body requirement of protein for an adult is about 1g/kg body weight. It is desirable that one fifth of this requirement should be animal protein.

Protein deficiency is related to amino acid deficiency and is accompanied by deficiency of minerals and vitamins. **Protein Calorie Malnutrition** (PCM) means deficiency of calories due to deficiency of protein. It is also known as **Protein Energy Malnutrition** (PEM).

A. Protein Deficiency Diseases

Diseases induced due to deficiency of protein are Kwashiorkor, Marasmus and Marasmic-Kwashiorkar.

(a) Kwashiorkar

Kwa means 'red boy'. It is a severe protein deficiency disease and is the most widespread deficiency disease of the world. Kwashiorkar is usually seen in the children between the age groups of 1 to 4 years. Kwashiorkar is common in Southern Mexico, Northern South America, Tropical Africa and India - all countries of low agricultural productivity. It is most common in poor rural children, displaced from the breast by the next child and given a very low protein starchy porridge.

Features

- Edema
- Hair pale and thinned
- Patches of pigmentation and desquamation on skin
- Moon face
- Palpable liver
- Will not eat

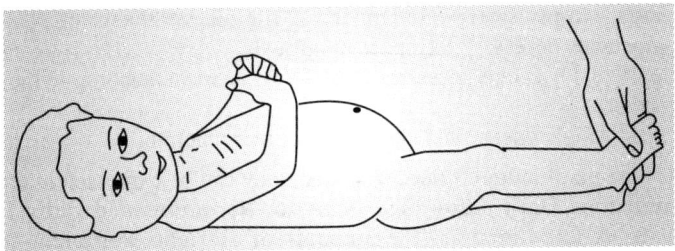

Fig. 2.2. Kwashiorkor.

Synthesis of two proteins made in the liver is reduced: (a) plasma albumin, hence edema, and (b) low density lipoproteins, hence lipids accumulate in the liver. Some of the features of kwashiorkor may be due to associated zinc deficiency. The principal clinical features include i) retarded growth, ii) anemia, iii) loss of appetite, iv) edema, v) diarrhoea, vi) scanty hair growth, vii) tissue swelling, viii) loss of pigmentation, and ix) apathy. Pure cases of Kwashiorkor can develop in a few weeks and the patients sometimes have normal weight for age. It is less common than Marasmus. Treatment consists of a diet comprised largely of dry skimmed milk. Improving the quantity and quality of proteins in the diet can prevent the disease.

(b) Marasmus

Nutritional marasmus is the commonest severe form of protein-energy malnutrition i.e. the childhood version of starvation, and involves lack of requisite calories needed by the body. It generally occurs in children between age groups of 0.5 to 5 years. This condition occurs at a younger age than Kwashiorkor. The characteristic syndromes include failure to gain weight, wasting of muscles and subcutaneous fat. The child is irritable but feels good appetite.

Features

- No edema
- Normal hair
- Grossly underweight
- Old man's face
- No body fat
- Gross muscle wasting

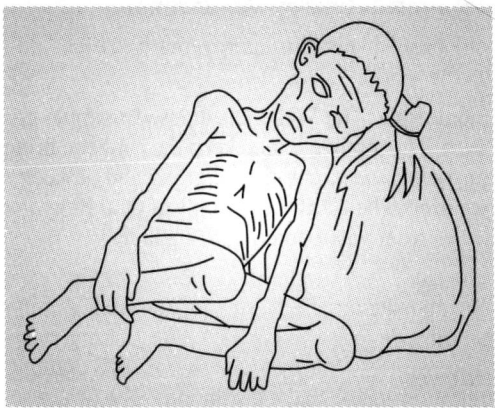

Fig. 2.3. Marasmus.

The cause of this condition is a diet very low in both calories and protein. Poor hygiene leads to gastroenteritis and a vicious circle starts. Diarrhoea leads to poor appetite and more dilute foods. In turn, further depletion leads to intestinal atrophy and more susceptibility to diarrhea.

(c) Marasmic-Kwashiorkor

Marasmic-Kwashiorkor has combined features of both Marasmus and Kwashiorkor conditions. Severe protein-energy malnutrition can be thought of as a spectrum from Marasmus to Kwashiorkor. Most affected children have some skin lesions, hair changes, and fatty liver (as in Kwashiorkor) together with the wasting of Marasmus. Malnourished children are likely to be depleted in other nutrients.

B. Treatment of Protein Deficiency Induced Diseases

The treatment of diseases induced by severe protein-energy malnutrition can be done in three phases-

    (a) Resuscitation: For correction of dehydration, electrolytes imbalance, acidosis, hypoglycemia, hypothermia, and the treatment of infections.

    (b) Start of cure: Re-feeding, gradually working up the calories (from 100 to 150 kcal per kg) and protein (to about 1.5 g per kg). There may be anorexia, and children often have to be hand fed, preferably in the lap of their mother or a nurse. Potassium, magnesium, zinc, and a multivitamin mixture are needed but iron should not be given for the first week.

    (c) Nutritional rehabilitation: After about three weeks if all goes well the child has lost edema and the skin is healed. The child is no longer ill and has a good appetite but is still underweight for age. It takes many weeks of good feeding for catch up growth to be complete. During this stage the child should be looked after in a convalescent home or by its mother, who should, if possible, have been educated about nutrition and provided with extra food. Locally available foods are best.

C. Prevention of Protein-Energy Malnutrition

Five measures to prevent protein-energy malnutrition are being actively promoted around the world.

(a) Growth monitoring: The WHO has devised a simple growth chart – the Road to Health card. The mother should keep the card and bring the child (plus card) to the nearest clinic regularly for weighing and advice.

(b) Oral rehydration: The UNICEF formula of Oral Rehydration Salt (ORS) is saving many lives from gastroenteritis. It includes:

Sodium chloride	3.5 g
Sodium bicarbonate	2.5 g
Potassium chloride	1.5 g
Glucose/sucrose	20 g/40 g
Clean drinking water to make a solution	1 litre

(c) Breast feeding is a matter of life and death in a poor community with no facilities for hygiene. Additional food, prepared from locally available products, is needed from four to six months of age.

(d) Immunization should be done against measles, tetanus, pertussis, diphtheria, polio, and tuberculosis.

(e) Family planning advice so that people can better take care of their children.

VITAMINS

Vitamins are complex substances that work as *regulators*. Often they act as *coenzymes*, or partners with enzymes, the proteins that cause reactions to take place in your body. Compared with carbohydrates, proteins, and fats; our body needs vitamins in only small amounts, hence they are called **micronutrients**. Vitamins do not supply energy directly. But they do regulate many processes that produce energy. Vitamins are themselves not synthesized by the body in sufficient amounts but they enable the body to use other nutrients.

These are organic compounds divided into two groups:

1. Fat-soluble vitamins
2. Water-soluble vitamins.

The category describes an important quality – how they are carried in food and transported in your body. As their name implies, fat-soluble vitamins (vitamins A, D, E, and K) dissolve in fat. Our body can store fat-soluble vitamins in body fat, so consuming too much of any fat-soluble vitamins for too long, usually from vitamin pills or other dietary supplements, can be harmful. Vitamins A and D, for example, can build up to toxic levels. High intakes of vitamins E and K usually are not linked to symptoms of toxicity. Water-soluble vitamins (B-complex vitamins and vitamin C) dissolve in water. For the most part, water-soluble vitamins are not stored in our body; at least not in significant amounts.

A. Fat-Soluble Vitamins

(a) Vitamin A

Functions

Vitamin A plays following vital functions:

1. It is necessary for normal bone growth and normal skin.
2. It promotes normal vision, and helps our eyes to see normally in the dark and helping to adjust for the lower level of light.
3. It promotes the growth and health of cells and tissues throughout our body; important for reproduction and development of the embryo.
4. It protects us from infections by keeping skin and tissues in our mouth, stomach, intestines, and respiratory, genital, and urinary tracts healthy.
5. It also works as an antioxidant in the form of carotenoids, and may reduce the risk for certain cancers and other diseases of aging.

Carotenoids are also thought to have health benefits beyond being precursors for vitamin A.

Deficiency

Symptoms of a significant deficiency of vitamin A include – eye problems; dry, scaly skin; problems with reproduction; and poor growth. The deficiency of vitamin A leads to night blindness, Bitot's spots, and keratomalacia. In vitamin A deficiency, there is metaplasia of conjunctival epithelium and loss of mucus production, leading to xerophthalmia. Other epithelia, like respiratory are similarly affected and their resistance to infection is lowered.

Over-consumption

Because it is stored in our body, large intakes of vitamin A, taken over time, can be quite harmful and may cause headache, liver damage, bone and joint pain, vomiting or appetite loss, abnormal bone growth, nerve damage, and birth defects. Beta carotene from fruits and vegetables is acceptable.

Daily requirement

From age 14 onward, the RDA is 900 micrograms Retinol Activity Equivalents (RAE) of vitamin A for males and 700 micrograms RAE for females. During pregnancy, the recommendation is 770 micrograms per day and during breast-feeding, 1200 micrograms RAE daily.

The tolerable upper intake limit is 2800 micrograms of RAEs daily for ages 14 to 18, and 3000 micrograms daily during adulthood. Retinol, beta carotene, and other pro-vitamin A carotenoids determine RAE.

Note: The RDAs (2001) measure vitamin A in Retinol Activity Equivalents (RAEs), reflecting retinol and carotenoid units. The quantity of vitamin A can be expressed in other ways: *International Units* (IU) – used for food labels and dietary supplements, or as *Retinol Equivalents* (RE) – used in the RDAs and many nutrient databases.

Vitamin A derived from animal based foods or supplements: 1 RE = 1 RAE
Vitamin A derived from Plant based foods: 1 RE = 2 RAE

Sources

Vitamin A comes from liver, fish oil, and eggs. Foods fortified with vitamin A – vanaspati, margarine, and milk are also important sources of this vitamin. Carotenoids, such as alpha carotene and beta carotene, come from foods of plant origin. Certain carotenoids are modified to form vitamin A (referred to as pro-vitamin A carotenoids) in our body. Carotenoids are found in red, yellow, orange, and many dark-green leafy vegetables. Plant sources of carotenoids are especially important to those who eat few animal based foods.

Marketed preparations of Vitamin A

Marketed preparation	Formulation	Manufacturer
Aro-G	Tablet	Geolife Sciences
Rovigon	Tablet	Nicholas
Vitriv-A	Tablet	East African
Wyamin	Capsule	Wyeth
Aquasol-A	Injection	USV

(b) Vitamin D

It is also known as the *Sunshine Vitamin*. Vitamin D_2 (calciferol) and vitamin D_3 (cholecalciferol) are nutritionally important forms of vitamin D.

Functions

It promotes the absorption of two minerals – calcium and phosphorus, in the formation of bones and teeth. It helps to deposit these minerals in bones and teeth, making them stronger and healthier and also regulates how much calcium should remain in our blood so additional vitamin D must be available through the diet in places where solar radiation is insufficient.

Deficiency

Children with a signicant vitamin D deficiency may develop rickets, or defective bone growth. Fortifying milk with vitamin D has virtually wiped out rickets in the United States. Rickets may, however, become a problem again if juice or soft drinks are consumed regularly in place of milk. Vitamin D deficiency is responsible for rickets in growing children and oesteomalacia in adults. Both diseases are common in India.

Over-consumption

Too much vitamin D can be toxic, possibly leading to kidney stones or damage, weak muscles and bones, excessive bleeding, and other problems.

Daily requirement

To maintain healthy bones, the guideline for vitamin D goes up to 10 micrograms, or 400 IU daily for adults over age 50. Over 70 years, the guideline increases to 15 micrograms, or 600 IU, per day. The daily requirements of vitamin D are 2.5 micrograms (100 IU) for adults, 5 micrograms (200 IU) for infants and children while 10 micrograms (400 IU) during pregnancy and lactation.

1 microgram cholecalciferol = 40 IU vitamin D

Sources

Our body can make vitamin D on exposure to sunlight, or ultraviolet light on the skin. To get enough vitamin D, it takes only 20 to 40 minutes of sun, three times a week, on our hands, arms, and face without sun screen. Darker skin needs more sun exposure; lighter skin, less. During the winter, and for older people whose skin is less efficient at converting sun exposure to vitamin D, milk is fortified with vitamin D. Vitamin D_2 may be derived from exposure to ultraviolet rays in sunlight. Vitamin D_3 is a naturally occurring substance found in sufficient amounts in egg yolk and fish liver oils and in small amounts in milk and butter. Cheese, some fish (like sardines and salmon), and fortified breakfast cereals and margarine also contain small amounts of vitamin D.

Marketed preparations of Vitamin D

Marketed preparation	Formulation	Manufacturer
Anca-D_3	Injection	Ancalima
Arachitol	Injection	Solvey
Corn D_3	Injection	Unicorn
Duracal	Injection	Ultramark H. Care
Apcical	Powder	Apids Pharma

(c) Vitamin E

It is a naturally occurring fat-soluble vitamin and occurs as alpha, beta, gamma and delta tocopherols.

Functions

1. Works as an antioxidant by preventing the oxidation of Low Density Lipids (LDL), cholesterol, and perhaps lowering the risk for heart disease and stroke. Its antioxidant activity also may help to reduce the risk of other health problems, such as some types of cancer.
2. As an antioxidant, it protects essential fatty acids and vitamin A.

Deficiency

Vitamin E is so abundant in food, a deficiency of vitamin E is rare.

Over-consumption

Eating plenty of vitamin E rich foods does not produce a problem. However, taking large doses of it as a dietary supplement appears to have no benefits and hence it is not recommended.

Daily requirement

The RDA guideline for males and females age 14 and over is 15 milligrams of alpha-tocopherol each day. Depending on their age children need less vitamin E. During pregnancy, women still need 15 mg daily; during breast-feeding the recommendation goes up to 19 mg daily.

Note: Vitamin E is a group of substances called tocopherols with different potencies. Alpha-tocopherol is its most potent form. On food and supplement labels, the amount is given in International Units (IU) of alpha-tocopherol, *not* in milligrams. Fifteen milligrams of alpha-tocopherol is equal to about 22 IU of d-alpha-tocopherol (natural vitamin E) and about 33 IU of dl-alpha-tocopherol (a synthetic form in fortified foods and some supplements). The "natural" form of vitamin E is more efficiently used than the synthetic form.

Sources

The richest sources of vitamin E are seed oils and oils of cereal germs. The best sources of vitamin E are vegetable oils for example, soybean, corn, cottonseed, and safflower. Nuts (especially almonds and hazelnuts), seeds (especially sunflower seeds), and wheat germ oil are also good sources. Green, leafy vegetables provide smaller amounts.

Marketed preparations of Vitamin E

Marketed preparation	*Formulation*	*Manufacturer*
Erovit Plus	Soft Gel Capsule	Royal Labs
Genac-200	Soft Gel Capsule	Genetic Pharma
Restofit	Capsule	Stedman Pharma
Bio-E	Capsule	Dr. Reddy's Lab
Elimcee	Capsule	Nicholas Piramal

(d) Vitamin K

It refers to a group of related compounds derived from menadione. Vitamin K_1 (phylloquinone) is found in plants. Vitamin K_2 (menaquinone-7) is synthesized by microorganisms and is found in animal tissues and bacteria. Vitamin K is stable to heat and exposure to air but is destroyed by light, strong acids, alkalis and oxidizing agents.

Functions

1. Vitamin K is necessary for normal blood coagulation. Synthesis of the four blood clotting factors, II, VII, IX and X is dependent on vitamin K.
2. It helps to make some proteins that cause our blood to coagulate, or form a clot, when there is bleeding. In this way, bleeding stops.
3. It also promotes the formation of some other body proteins for our blood, bones, and kidneys.

Deficiency

Deficiency of vitamin K causes hypoprothrombinaemia. Blood does not coagulate normally and therefore blood-clotting time is significantly prolonged. This further leads to hemorrhages.

Over-consumption

No symptoms have been observed but control is still the best approach. People taking blood thinning drugs, or anti-coagulants, need to eat foods with vitamin K in moderation.

Daily requirement

The daily requirement for an adult is 0.03 mg/kg body weight. During adulthood the intake goes up i.e. 120 micrograms and 90 micrograms daily for men and women, respectively. The recommendations remain the same during pregnancy or breast-feeding. To make sure infants have enough, newborns typically receive a shot of vitamin K.

Sources

Like vitamin D, our body can produce vitamin K on its own from certain bacteria in our intestines. The best food sources are green leafy vegetables such as spinach and broccoli. However, a variety of foods, milk and other dairy foods, meat, eggs, cereal, fruits, and other vegetables provide smaller amounts.

Marketed preparations of Vitamin K

Marketed preparation	Formulation	Manufacturer
Styptindon	Tablet	Indo Pharma
Cadisper-C	Tablet	Cadila
K-Win	Injection	Mercury
Kapilin	Injection	Galxo-Smithkline

B. Water-Soluble Vitamins

(a) Vitamin B₁ (Thiamine)

Functions

1. Thiamine functions as a coenzyme in energy metabolism or utilization of carbohydrates.
2. It is essential in the synthesis of pentoses and NADPH (Nicotinamide adenine dinucleotide phosphate).
3. It is also involved in nerve impulse transmission.

Deficiency

The principal thiamine deficiency disease is *beri-beri*. It is classified into dry, wet and infantile *beri-beri*. *Dry beri-beri* is characterized by peripheral polyneuritis, paralysis and muscle atrophy. *Wet beri-beri* is characterized by congestive heart failure with cardiac dilatation, damage of the cardiac musculature, serous effusions and edema. Infantile *beri-beri* is the leading cause of infant mortality in many developing areas of the world. *Beri-beri* can be eliminated by taking thiamine rich foods and stopping all alcohol. Generally thiamine deficiency affects the cardiovascular, muscular, nervous and gastro-intestinal systems.

Daily requirement

The RDA for thiamine is tied to our energy needs: 1.2 mg daily for males age 14 through adulthood. For females, the recommendation is 1 mg daily from ages 14 -18 and 1.1 mg daily from age 19 onwards. During pregnancy and breast-feeding, the recommended amount may go up to 1.4 mg daily.

Sources

It is present in cereals, pulses, nuts and yeasts. Whole-grain and enriched grain products such as bread, rice, pasta, tortillas, and fortified cereals provide much of the required thiamine. Pork, liver, and other organ meats provide signicant amounts of thiamine. It is also present in small amounts in milk and vegetables.

Marketed preparations of Vitamin B₁ (Thiamine)

Marketed preparation	Formulation	Manufacturer
Therabine	Injection	Parex Pharma
Tim	Injection	Gentech H. Care
Benalgis	Tablet	Franco-Indian

(b) Vitamin B₂ (Riboflavin)

Functions

1. It helps to produce energy in all cells of our body.
2. It helps in conversion of tryptophan amino acid in our food into niacin.

Deficiency

Riboflavin deficiency is common in India. It is characterized by cheilosis, angular stomatitis, glossitis, seborrheic dermatitis, scrotal deformities and ocular manifestations like corneal vascularization, photophobia, itching, burning and circumcorneal capillary engorgement. Deficiency symptoms also include eye disorders (including cataracts), dry and flaky skin and a sore, red tongue.

Over-consumption

No problem reported.

Daily requirement

Like thiamine, the RDA for riboflavin is tied to our energy needs. Adult men need 1.3 mg daily and adult women need 1.1 mg daily. During pregnancy, the recommendation is 1.4 mg and during breast-feeding, the amount goes up to 1.6 mg daily.

Sources

Milk and other dairy foods are major sources of riboflavin. Some organ meats like liver, kidney, and heart are also excellent sources. Enriched bread and other grain products, eggs, green leafy vegetables, and nuts supply smaller amounts. Riboflavin content of pulses and cereals can be increased by germination.

Note: Since sunlight (ultraviolet light) destroys riboflavin, milk should be packed in opaque plastic or cardboard containers, not in clear glass containers.

Marketed preparations of Vitamin B_2

Marketed preparation	Formulation	Manufacturer
Riboflavin	Tablet	Shraya
Anvit Fort	Capsule	Anrose Pharma
Retolbid	Capsule	East African

(c) Niacin

It is also known as nicotinic acid. Niacin is readily converted to niacinamide (nicotinamide) in human. Strictly speaking niacin is not a vitamin as it may be synthesized endogenously from the essential amino acid, tryptophan in the presence of vitamin B_6 as pyridoxal phosphate. Sixty milligrams of tryptophan provide 1 mg of niacin. Niacin intake is therefore expressed in terms of niacin equivalents (NE) where:

    1 NE = 1 mg niacin (nicotinic acid) = 60 mg tryptophan

Functions

1. Niacin, in the form of nicotinic acid, reduces hyperlipidemia, since it reduces LDL cholesterol (bad cholesterol) and increases HDL cholesterol (good cholesterol).
2. It is essential for the metabolism of carbohydrates, fats and proteins.
3. It is required for the normal functioning of skin, intestinal and nervous systems.
4. It helps the enzymes to function normally in body.
3. It helps produce energy in all the cells of our body.

Deficiency

Niacin deficiency can lead to nutritional disease called *pellagra,* which presents as the **4 D's** – *dermatitis, diarrhoea, dementia and death.* Early signs of niacin deficiency include fatigue, anorexia, weakness, mild gastrointestinal disturbance, anxiety, irritability and depression. A scaly, bilateral, pigmented dermatitis appears generally in areas exposed to sunlight. Niacin deficiency can be overcome by the consumption of a good mixed diet containing milk and/or meat. For people who consume adequate amounts of protein-rich foods, a niacin deficiency is not likely.

Over-consumption

Consuming excessive amounts, likely from a dietary supplement, may cause flushed skin, rashes, or liver damage.

Daily requirement

Niacin recommendations are given in Niacin Equivalents (NE). Like thiamine and riboflavin, its recommendation is tied to energy needs. The advice for adult males is 16 mg NE daily, and for adult females, 14 mg NE daily. During pregnancy, 18 mg NE is advised and during breast-feeding, 17 mg NE daily.

Sources

High protein foods are typically good sources of niacin like poultry, fish, beef, peanut, butter, and legumes. Niacin is also added to many enriched and fortified grain products.

Marketed preparations of Niacin

Marketed preparation	Formulation	Manufacturer
Basiton Forte	Tablet	Nicholas Piramal
Becosules	Capsule	Pfizer
Betonin	Elixer	Abbott

(d) Vitamin B₆

It refers to three pyridines: pyridoxine, pyridoxal and pyridoxamine. These compounds are closely related and are converted to the biologically active coenzyme form of pyridoxal phosphate. In animal products, vitamin B_6 is found largely as pyridoxal and pyridoxamine. In plants the main form of vitamin B_6 is pyridoxine.

Functions

1. It is important in metabolism of amino acids, fats and carbohydrates.
2. It helps our body to make non-essential amino acids, or protein components, which are then used to make body cells.
3. It helps in conversion of tryptophan amino acid into two important body substances: niacin and serotonin.
4. It helps to produce other body chemicals, including insulin, hemoglobin, and antibodies that fight infection.

Deficiency

Vitamin B_6 deficiency is associated with peripheral neuritis and can cause mental convulsions among infants, depression, nausea, or greasy, flaky skin. Pyridoxine deficiency is rare because balanced diet usually contains this vitamin.

For infants, breast milk and properly prepared infant formulas contain enough vitamin B_6.

Over-consumption

Large doses, taken over time, can cause nerve damage.

Daily requirement

The RDA is 1.3 mg daily for adult males and females upto age 50 years. After age 50, the RDA increases to 1.7 mg daily for males and 1.5 mg for females. The amount increases to 1.9 mg daily during pregnancy and 2.0 mg daily during breast-feeding.

Sources

Chicken, fish, pork, liver, and kidney are the best sources of vitamin B_6. Green vegetables, whole grains, nuts, bran of cereals and legumes also supply reasonable amounts of it.

Marketed preparations of Vitamin B_6

Marketed preparation	Formulation	Manufacturer
Folikit	Tablet	Unique Life Sciences
Spera 69	Tablet	Indoco

(e) Pantothenic acid

Functions

1. Pantothenic acid is a component of coenzyme-A which functions in acyl transfer reactions of the citric acid (Krebs) cycle.
2. It helps our body cells to produce energy.
3. It helps to metabolize or use proteins, and carbohydrates from food.
4. It is also involved in the metabolism of lipids and in the synthesis of steroids.

Deficiency

Dietary deficiency of pantothenic acid is rare in healthy people. Symptoms of its deficiency are abdominal pain and soreness, nausea, personality changes, insomnia, impaired adrenal function, weakness and cramps in the legs, paresthesia of the hands and feet and impaired antibody production

Over-consumption

Occasional diarrhoea and water retention.

Daily requirement

The AI (Adequate Intake) for pantothenic acid is 5 mg daily for ages 14-18 and for adults. During pregnancy and breast-feeding, the AI increases to 6 and 7 mg, respectively.

Sources

It is widely available in food. Meat, poultry, fish, whole-grain cereals, and legumes are among the better sources. Milk, vegetables, and fruits also contain varying amounts.

Marketed preparations of Pantothenic acid (Vitamin B₅) as Calcium Pantothenate

Marketed preparation	Formulation	Manufacturer
Lactocom Forti	Capsule	Cadila
Livobion	Capsule	Pharmasynth
Macro-Z	Capsule	Intas Remedies
Manavite	Capsule	Wyeth
Mittavin	Capsule	Nicholas Piramal
Jolvit	Tablet	Geolife Sciences
Mutineuron Forte	Tablet	Bestochem
O-Vit	Tablet	Oscar Remedies
Optineuron	Tablet	Lupin
Supradyn	Tablet	Nicholas

(f) Folic acid

Folic acid occurs either as free or bound folate form.

Functions

1. It plays an essential role in making new body cells by helping to produce DNA and RNA.
2. It works with vitamin B_{12} to form hemoglobin in red blood cells.
3. It may help to protect against heart disease.
4. It helps to lower the risk of delivering a baby with neural tube defects such as spina bifida, and it helps to control plasma homocysteine levels, which is associated with increased risk of cardiovascular disease.

Deficiency

Folate deficiency may occur from a poor diet. A deficiency affects normal cell division and protein synthesis, especially impairing growth. Pregnant women, who don't get enough folate, especially during the first trimester, have a greater risk of delivering a baby with neural tube defects such as spina bifida (the neural tube in an embryo becomes the spinal cord and brain). To reduce risk, all women of child-bearing age should consume adequate amounts. Severe deficiency of folate may cause infertility or even sterility.

Over-consumption

Over-consumption can mask a vitamin B_{12} deficiency and may interfere with certain medications. Taking excess amounts as a dietary supplement offers no known benefits.

Daily requirement

For folate, the RDA for males from age 14 through adulthood is 400 micrograms daily. Women capable of becoming pregnant (14 to 50 years) should get 400 micrograms of folic acid daily from fortified foods, vitamin supplements, or a combination of the two, in addition to the folate found naturally in certain foods. Pregnancy increases the recommended amount to 600 micrograms daily and during breast-feeding, 500 micrograms are advised.

Sources

It is present in large amounts in fresh green leafy vegetables, cauliflower, liver, kidney and yeast. Orange juice, lentils, dried beans, spinach, broccoli, peanuts, and avocados are among the good sources of naturally occurring folate. Enriched grain products – such as most of breads, flour, crackers, corn grits, cornmeal, farina, rice, macaroni, and noodles – must be fortified with folic acid. It is also synthesized by intestinal bacteria. Most of the folic acid is destroyed during cooking.

Marketed preparations of Folic acid

Marketed preparation	Formulation	Manufacturer
Alfolic	Injection	Altak Pharma
BFA	Tablet	Bionet India
FH-12	Tablet	Bestochem
Feed	Tablet	Santo Formulations
Fol 5	Tablet	German Remedies
Folvite	Tablet	Wyeth
Folinal	Tablet	Alembic
Forich	Tablet	Zee Lab
Vacofol	Tablet	Sandoz

(g) Vitamin B_{12}

Cyanocobalamin or vitamin B_{12} is water-soluble and synthesized exclusively by microorganisms.

Functions

1. It works closely with folate to make red blood cells.

2. It serves as a vital part of many body chemicals and so occurs in each body cell.
3. It helps our body to use fatty acids and some amino acids.

Deficiency

It is mainly stored in liver in coenzyme forms and hence deficiency is rare. Deficiency of vitamin B_{12} causes megaloblastic anemia and may also result in fatigue, nerve damage, a smooth tongue, or very sensitive skin. Nutritional Megaloblastic Anemia (NMA) is common in India. Foods fortified with vitamin B_{12} or dietary supplements can prevent vitamin B_{12} deficiency.

A deficiency of vitamin B_{12} can also be masked, if extra folic acid is taken to treat or prevent anemia. People who develop pernicious anemia miss a body chemical called **intrinsic factor**. This problem can be medically treated with injections of vitamin B_{12}.

Over-consumption

No symptoms are known, but taking extra vitamin B_{12} to boost energy has no basis.

Daily requirement

The RDA is 2.4 micrograms daily for adults. The recommendation increases to 2.6 micrograms daily during pregnancy and 2.8 micrograms daily during breast-feeding.

Sources

It is present in large amounts in animal products, liver, kidney, meat, eggs, fish, yeast, milk and cheese. It is also synthesized by bacteria in colon.

Marketed preparation of Vitamin B_{12}

Marketed preparation	Formulation	Manufacturer
Siocobin	Injection	Albert David

(h) Vitamin C (Ascorbic acid)

Functions

1. It works as an antioxidant to inhibit damage to body cells.
2. It helps in the formation of collagen, or the intracellular cement substance, which is necessary for body growth, tissue repair and wound healing.
3. It helps to keep capillary walls and blood vessels firm, and so protects our body from bruising.
4. It helps our body to absorb iron and copper from plant sources of food.
5. It helps to keep our gums healthy.
6. It helps in the synthesis of adrenaline and hydrocortisone.
7. It protects us from infection by stimulating the formation of antibodies, which boost our body immunity.

8. Vitamin C may also play a role in membrane permeability, leukocyte function and prevention of accumulation of histamine in the body.
9. Roles of ascorbic acid in prevention of common cold and protection against infection are yet to be proved scientifically.

Deficiency

A severe deficiency of vitamin C leads to scurvy, which is characterized by weakness, spongy and bleeding gums (scorbutic gum), loose teeth, resorbed dentine. Its deficiency also causes hemorrhages in skin and other hemorrhages. Wounds may not heal properly either. Because vitamin C rich foods are widely available, so its deficiency is no longer a common deficiency.

Over-consumption

Since vitamin C is water-soluble, our body excretes the excess. Very large doses may cause kidney stones and/or diarrhoea, and for those with iron overload, excessive vitamin C (which enhances iron absorption) can make the problem worse.

Daily requirement

The RDA for females and males ages 14–18 is 65 mg and 75 mg of vitamin C daily, respectively. Adult males need 90 mg daily; adult females, 75 mg of vitamin C daily for everyday needs (about the amount in 3/4 cup of orange juice). Women need somewhat more during pregnancy (80 to 85 mg) and breast-feeding (115 to 120 mg). For people who smoke, the RDA for vitamin C is increased by 35 mg daily to counteract the oxidative damage from nicotine.

Sources

Vitamin C mainly comes from plant sources of food. All citrus fruits, including oranges, grapefruits, and tangerines, are good sources. *Amla* is one of the richest sources of ascorbic acid. Many other fruits and vegetables, including berries, melons, peppers, fresh green and leafy vegetables, potatoes and tomatoes also supply signicant amounts.

Marketed preparations of Vitamin C

Marketed preparation	Formulation	Manufacturer
Celin	Tablet	Glaxo-Smithkline
Cell-C, Limcee	Tablet	Nicholas Piramal
Chewcee	Tablet	Wyeth
Solcee-Z	Tablet	Alchemist
Vitriv-C	Tablet	East African
Redoxon	Tablet	Nicholas

(i) Biotin

Functions

1. It helps our body to produce energy in cells.
2. It helps to metabolize (or use) proteins, fats, and carbohydrates from food.

Deficiency

That's rarely a problem for healthy people who eat a healthy diet because the body also produces biotin from intestinal bacteria.

Over-consumption

Not reported.

Daily requirement

The Adequate Intake (AI) for biotin is 30 micrograms daily for adult males and females, including during pregnancy. The AI increases to 35 micrograms daily during breast-feeding.

Sources

Biotin is found in a wide variety of foods. Eggs, liver, yeast breads, and cereals are among the best sources.

Marketed preparations of Biotin

Marketed preparation	Formulation	Manufacturer
Apotin	Tablet	Apotex Lifesciences
Axytin	Tablet	Axyzen
Beten Forte	Tablet	Dr. Derma
Wintin	Tablet	Dermawin
Oktin	Tablet	Wel 'N' Drugs
Weltin	Capsule	Articon Labs

MINERALS

A number of minerals are essential for body functions. They are classified as *macro*minerals or *micro*minerals (trace elements) depending on their dietary requirement. The macrominerals include calcium, phosphorus, potassium, sodium, chloride, sulfur and magnesium. The trace elements include copper, cobalt, chromium, fluorine, iodine, iron, manganese, molybdenum, nickel, selenium, silicon, tin, vanadium and zinc. Minerals may function as co-factors of enzymes, as components of organic compounds and as structural components of bones and teeth and are catalysts for many biological processes. Minerals may also participate in contraction and conduction of nerve impulses.

Table 2.1. Recommended vitamins intake for individuals

Age group (years)	A (µg/d)	C (µg/d)	D (µg/d)	E (µg/d)	K (µg/d)	Thiamine (mg/d)	Riboflavin (mg/d)	Niacin (mg/d)	B_6 (mg/d)	B_{12} (µg/d)	Folic acid (µg/d)	Biotin (µg/d)
						Males						
19-70	900	90	5	15	120	1.2	1.3	16	1.3	2.4	400	30
						Females						
19-70	700	75	5	15	90	1.1	1.1	14	1.3	2.4	400	30
						Pregnancy						
19-50	770	85	5	15	90	1.4	1.4	18	1.9	2.6	600	30
						Lactation						
19-50	1300	120	5	19	90	1.4	1.6	17	2.0	2.8	500	35

A. Macrominerals

(a) Calcium

Calcium is the most abundant cation in the human body. The body of an adult usually contains about 1200 g of calcium. More than 99% of the calcium is present in bones and teeth. The remaining 1% of total body calcium is necessary for a variety of metabolic processes including enzyme activation, hormone function, nerve transmission, muscle contraction, blood clotting and membrane transport.

Sources

Milk and milk products are the richest dietary sources of calcium. Lesser amounts of calcium are found in shellfish, egg yolk, canned sardines and salmon (with bones), soybeans and certain green leafy vegetables such as spinach, turnip and mustard greens, broccoli and kale. As a result of fortification, infant cereals are excellent sources of calcium. More recently, the fortification of foods such as orange juice and flour has become additional sources of calcium in the diet. In hard water areas, drinking water may also be a significant source.

Deficiency

Indian diets are poor in calcium. Calcium deficiency may occur in infants who are breast fed by mothers suffering from vitamin D deficiency. Calcium deficiency may occur in pregnant and lactating women. Low dietary calcium intake may produce rickets and osteomalacia. Severe calcium deficiency in children may also result in stunted growth, muscle weakness, parathyroid hyperplasia, hyperirritability, tetany and death.

(b) Magnesium

The human body contains 20 to 28 g of magnesium. About 55% is present in bone while 27% is found in muscles. The remainder is found in the cells and extracellular fluids. Magnesium performs a vital role in the enzymatic reactions involving ATP. It is needed for the activation of thiokinases used in fatty acid oxidation as well as amino acid acyl synthetases. Magnesium is required for protein synthesis. It plays a role in maintenance of cell membranes and neuromuscular transmission.

Sources

Magnesium occurs widely in foods, particularly those of plant origin. Sources include green vegetables (magnesium is a component of chlorophyll), cereals, grains, meat, milk, seafood, cocoa and nuts. Plasma magnesium concentrations range from 2 to 3 mg/dL.

Deficiency

Due to the abundance of magnesium in the food supply, primary magnesium deficiency is rare. Magnesium deficiency results in hypocalcemia and hypokalemia. Its deficiency affects the gastrointestinal, neuromuscular, cardiovascular and hematologic systems. Dysphagia, anemia, cardiac arrhythmias, tremors, weakness, failure to thrive and psychiatric disturbances may be present. Magnesium deficiency ultimately results in tachycardia, fibrillations, convulsions and death.

(c) Phosphorous

The phosphorus content of an adult man is approximately 700 g. About 80% of the body's phosphorus is found in bone as calcium phosphate and hydroxyapatite. In the bone the phosphorus to calcium ratio is 1:2. There is no free elemental phosphorus in the body. It is present as a constituent of various lipids, proteins, carbohydrates, enzymes, nucleic acid and ATP (adenosine tri phosphate). In its ionic form, phosphorus serves to modify acid-base balance in the blood. Phosphorus acts as a co-factor in a number of enzyme systems involved in carbohydrate, protein and fat metabolism. Phosphorus is important as a component of phospholipids in cell membranes, lipoproteins, etc, and is involved in the renal excretion of hydrogen ions.

Sources

Protein foods of animal origin such as meat, fish, poultry and eggs are excellent sources of phosphorus. Milk and cheese are good sources of phosphorus.

Deficiency

Phosphorus deficiency has been reported in individuals consuming a prolonged and excessive intake of non-absorbable antacids, which bind dietary phosphorus preventing its absorption. Symptoms of phosphorus deficiency include weakness, anorexia, malaise and pain in the bones. Hemolytic anemia, granulocyte dysfunction, erythrocyte glycolysis, neurologic and psychiatric disorders, hypercalciuria and renal calculi may also result from phosphorus deficiency.

(d) Sodium & Potassium

Sodium and potassium are essential for normal growth and body functions. Sodium is the predominant extracellular electrolyte and potassium is the major intracellular cation. They are both involved in regulating water- and acid-base balance, in membrane permeability, nerve conduction and muscle action. Changes in extracellular sodium concentration can affect arterial pressure whereas changes in blood potassium concentration can affect cardiac performance.

Sources

Sodium and potassium are widely distributed in foods. Dietary sources of sodium include table salt (sodium chloride) and sodium-based food additives used in commercially processed and cured foods. Foods that have relatively high levels of naturally occurring sodium include milk and milk products, meat, fish (particularly ocean fish), seafood, poultry and eggs. Good sources of potassium are meat, poultry, fish, organ meats, milk and milk products and certain fruits and vegetables. High potassium fruits include avocado, banana, apricot, dried fruits, melons and oranges. Some high potassium vegetables are broccoli, brussels sprouts, parsnips, squash, potatoes, dry beans and peas.

Deficiency

Deficiency of both sodium and potassium under ordinary conditions is virtually unknown. However, in excessive sweat loss, severe vomiting and diarrhoea, and in renal pathology; depletion of sodium can result in muscular cramps, mental confusion, apathy, anorexia and coma. Potassium depletion, which occurs when using diuretics, will cause muscular weakness, cardiac arrhythmia and mental confusion.

B. Trace Elements

(a) Fluoride

Traces of fluoride are normally present in human tissues, notably in the bones, teeth, thyroid gland and skin. Fluoride is essential for the normal mineralization of bones and formation of dental enamel. The primary significance of this element in human nutrition is in the prevention of dental caries. Fluoride reduces the risk of dental decay.

Drinking water should usually contain 1 ppm of fluorine. Less than 0.5 ppm of fluorine in water leads to dental carries whereas excessive amounts lead to endemic fluoresces.

Sources

Most human adults ingest between 2 and 3 mg of fluorine daily. The chief source is usually drinking water, which, if it contains 1 ppm of fluorine, will supply 1 to 2 mg/day and will confer optimal protection against tooth decay. Compared with this source, the fluoride in foodstuffs is of little importance. Very few foods contain more than 1 ppm; the exception is sea fish, which may contain relatively large amounts in the order of 5 to 10 ppm. Another significant source is tea, particularly Chinese tea, which in the dry state, may contain as much as 100 ppm. In Britain and Australia, where tea is a popular beverage, the adult intake from this source may be as much as 1 mg daily.

Commercial baby foods generally contain less than 0.1 ppm fluoride. A significant source of fluoride for pre-school children is fluorinated toothpaste. As the practice of tooth brushing becomes more widespread among pre-school children, as many as 75% of children may be using toothpaste by 18 months of age.

The Committee on Nutrition of the American Academy of Pediatrics recommends that infants in non-fluorinated areas (water less than 0.3 ppm) be given a fluoride supplement from about 2 weeks of age. The dosage depends on the concentration of fluoride in the local drinking water.

(b) Iodine

Iodine is essential for all animals, including humans. Iodine is required as a component of the thyroid hormones thyroxine (T_4) and triiodothyronine (T_3).

Thyroxine and triiodothyronine are required for normal energy metabolism, thermoregulation, intermediary metabolism, protein synthesis, reproduction, growth, physical and mental development, hematopoiesis and neuromuscular function. The adult human body contains 10-20 mg iodine. About 70-80% of the iodine is concentrated in the thyroid gland. The remainder is distributed throughout the body with higher concentrations occurring in the salivary and gastric glands as well as in the dense connective tissue.

Sources

The best sources of iodine are seafood and seaweed, which are of limited significance in Western diets. Meat, milk and eggs may also provide iodine, their iodine content is influenced by the iodine provided in the animal feed. Soils of coastal areas are rich in iodine. Food fortification with iodine has been most effective in the eradication of iodine deficiency. In Canada, table salt must contain 0.01 percent potassium iodide. In the United States, where non-iodized salt is also available, iodized salt contains 76 microgram iodine per gram of salt. Since the introduction of iodized salt, goiter resulting from iodine deficiency has been virtually eliminated. Certain foods such as cabbage, rutabaga, and other members of the Brassica family contain *goitrogens,* which interfere with thyroid hormone synthesis. The uptake, synthesis and release of iodine by the thyroid gland is stimulated by thyroid stimulating hormone (TSH) released by the anterior pituitary gland.

Deficiency

Iodine deficiency is the most common cause of endemic goiter and cretinism in the world. Endemic goiter is one of the most prevalent nutritional deficiency problems that afflict millions of people in many parts of the world. Iodine deficiency results in enlargement of the thyroid gland (goiter). Severe iodine deficiency can produce myxedema, which is characterized by a dry, waxy type swelling, with abnormal deposits of mucoproteins under the skin.

Toxicity

Excessive dietary intake of iodine results in inhibition of thyroid hormone synthesis clinically known as the *Wolff-Chaikoff effect.* Generally, the body will adapt to the higher intake but in a few individuals the effect continues and the individual develops goiter. Hyperthyroidism resulting from excessive iodine intake is characterized by increased basal metabolism, goiter and disturbances in the autonomic nervous systems causing hyperirritability and increased creatinine metabolism.

(c) Iron

Iron is an essential element in all cells of the body. It plays a key role in oxygen transport and cellular respiration as a constituent of hemoglobin, myoglobin and the enzymes – cytochrome oxidase, peroxidase and catalase. Iron in the cellular cytochrome system is required for energy metabolism. In the adult male, total body iron amounts to 3.5 to 5.0 g. In the premenopausal woman approximately 2.5 g of iron is normally present.

Sources

The following are some good sources of iron: liver, heart, kidney, red meats, shell fish, egg yolk, dried beans, other legumes, dried fruits, nuts, green leafy vegetables, dark molasses and whole grain cereals. Iron-fortified cereal and cereal products such as flour, bread, infant- and breakfast cereals are also good sources when consumed as a dietary staple. Cow's milk is a poor source of iron as the iron in milk is poorly absorbed. Although breast milk supplies only about 0.5 to 0.8 mg of iron per day, the bioavailability of its iron is high. Normally, an infant born with an adequate store of iron will receive sufficient iron from breast milk in the first 4 to 6 months of life. Thereafter, additional sources such as iron-fortified infant cereals and other iron-rich baby foods are required.

Deficiency

Iron deficiency is one of the most prevalent nutritional problems in the world. Vegetable diets in India are mostly poor in iron content. The populations most susceptible to iron deficiency problem are infants and young children, menstruating females, pregnant women and individuals on energy restricted diets and older people. Iron deficiency leads to anemia i.e. reduction in the hemoglobin content of RBCs. Hemoglobin contains iron and hence deficiency of iron in diet causes a deficiency in hemoglobin content. Hemoglobin carries oxygen in the blood and therefore in iron deficiency anemia oxygen reduction in the blood causes sluggishness and fatigue and diminishes work and physical performance.

Iron deficiency is characterized by weakness, fatigue, poor work performance and changes in behavior.

Table 2.2. Recommended minerals intake for individuals

Age group (Years)	Ca (mg/d)	Mg (mg/d)	P (mg/d)	F (mg/d)	I (µg/d)	Fe (mg/d)
Children						
1–3	500	80	460	0.7	90	7
4–8	800	130	500	1	90	10
Male						
19–70	1000	400	700	4	150	8
Female						
19–70	1000	310	700	3	150	18

Toxicity

Excessive iron ingestion may result in hemosiderosis or deposition of iron in the tissues without harmful effect. Prolonged excessive intake may result in hemochromatosis in which further iron storage results in tissue damage, particularly the liver and the pancreas. Hyperpigmentation of the skin is another feature of this disorder.

The requirement of nutrients for pregnant and lactating women is usually greater. Similarly these requirements also vary according to age group like infants, children, adolescents and adults.

Marketed preparations containing different minerals

Marketed preparation	Formulation	Manufacturer
Sandocal Plus	Tablet	Novartis
Ossidos-T	Tablet	Wockhardt
Theragran-M	Tablet	Nicholas Piramal
Vistamina	Tablet	Medley
Prenatal	Capsule	Wyeth
Uni-OX	Capsule	Unicorn
V-Mix	Capsule	Chemo Drugs
Macalvit	Syrup	Novartis
Zingicare	Liquid	Medizone
Polybion	Injection	Merck

Fortunately several marketed formulations containing multivitamins plus minerals are available which meet the nutritional requirement of both, vitamins as well as minerals. Such preparations are easier to administer and hence have better compliance. Drops and syrups are particularly useful in children.

Marketed preparations containing Multivitamins + Minerals

Marketed preparation	Formulation	Manufacturer
ABCD	Drop	Geneka Biotech
Diakair	Syrup	PDC H. Care
Kenimix	Syrup	Kendall H. Care
Mmg	Syrup	Amro Pharma
Emrovit	Capsule	Mits H. Care

(Contd.)

Marketed preparation	Formulation	Manufacturer
Garner	Capsule	Affy Pharma
Regain	Capsule	JVD
Menal	Tablet	Esskay Bee Pharma
Provit	Tablet	Hitech Formulation
Retivit	Tablet	Shree Raj Pharma

BALANCED DIET

The main purpose of food consumed by human beings is to provide energy for growth, maintenance of body functions, and work. This energy is obtained from carbohydrates, fats and protein.

A **diet** is the kind of food on which a person or group lives. A **balanced diet** is one that contains a variety of foods in such quantity and proportion as to meet the need for energy, amino acids, vitamins, minerals, fats, carbohydrates and other nutrients; to maintain health, vitality and general well-being and also makes a small provision for extra nutrients to withstand short duration of leanness. A balanced diet is a means of protecting the population from nutritional deficiencies.

Any balanced diet should meet (i) the daily requirement of proteins (equivalent to 15-20% of daily energy intake), (ii) fat requirement (equivalent to 20-30% of daily energy intake), (iii) carbohydrates, rich in natural fibre to contribute to remaining food energy, and (iv) the requirement of micronutrients.

Table 2.3. Balanced diet formulated by ICMR

Food item (g)	Adult man (moderate work)	Adult woman (moderate work)	Children (1–3 yr.)	Boys (10–12 yr.)	Girls (10–12 yr.)
Cereals	520	440	175	420	380
Pulses*	50	45	35	45	45
Leafy vegetables	70	40	20	50	50
Roots and Tubers	60	50	10	30	30
Milk	200	150	300	250	250
Oil and Fat	45	25	15	40	35
Sugar or Jaggery	35	20	30	45	45

* *In case of non-vegetarians 50% of pulses can be substituted by (i) one egg or 30 g of meat or fish, (ii) additional 5 g of fat or oil; 100% of pulses can be substituted by (i) two eggs or 50 g of meat or fish, (ii) additional 10 g of fat or oil.*

Dietary preference of individuals, groups, communities etc are variable according to local economy, culture, taste, habits, religions, customs, climatic conditions etc. Balance diet formulated by Indian Council of Medical Research (ICMR) is given in Table 2.3.

A balanced diet containing all the essential nutrients can prevent most of the nutritional deficiency diseases. In this context a community pharmacist can play a key role in educating the general public about different aspects of nutrition and health.

3

Demography and Family Planning

INTRODUCTION

Control of human population is a major problem in India and most of the other countries of the world. Increasing population is the major obstacle in the all round development of our country. One of the measures to check the growing population is family planning. Pharmacists deal directly with the public and hence they are in a better position to educate the people about the hazards of unchecked population growth, importance of family planning and family planning methods.

DEMOGRAPHY

Demography is the scientific study of human population. It is mainly concerned with (*i*) change in population size, (*ii*) composition of the population, and (*iii*) the distribution of population. These three phenomenons are related to fertility, mortality, marriage, migration and social mobility; commonly known as **demographic processes**. The process of complete counting of all individuals in a country on a fixed date is known as **census**. In India first census took place in 1881 and the last in 2011. It is being conducted once in every 10 years ending with the digit 1. Hence next census shall be due in 2021.

The demographics of India are inclusive of the second most populous country in the world, with over 1.21 billion people (2011 census), more than one sixth of the world's population (Table 3.1). Its population growth rate is 1.41%, ranking 102nd in the world in 2010. India has more than 50% of its population below the age of 25 and more than 65% below the age of 35. It is expected that in 2020, the average age of an Indian will be 69 years, compared to 37 for China and 48 for Japan.

Table 3.1. Demography of India at a glance

Population	1,210,193,422 (estimated in 2011)
Growth rate	1.41% (estimated in 2009)
Birth rate	22.22 births/1,000 population (estimated in 2009)
Death rate	6.4 deaths/1,000 population (estimated in 2009)
Life expectancy	69.89 years (estimated in 2009)
Male	67.46 years (estimated in 2009)
Female	72.61 years (estimated in 2009)
Fertility rate	2.5 children born/woman (estimated in 2010)
Infant mortality rate	30.15 deaths/1,000 live births (estimated in 2009)

DEMOGRAPHY CYCLE

History of population of any country follows a definite pattern called demographic cycle, which consists of five stages.

(a) **First stage:** This is a stationary phase in which high birth rate and high death rates nullify each other. Thus the population remains stationary. First stage is also called *high stationary stage*. Till 1920 India remained in the first stage.

(b) **Second stage:** This stage is characterized by an increase in population. The birth rate remains unchanged but the death rate declines. Hence second stage is also called as *early expanding stage*. Many countries in Africa and South Asia are in this phase.

(c) **Third Stage:** It is also known as *late expanding stage* characterized by continued decline of the death rate but the birth rate also tends to fall. Total population shows increase because total births exceed total deaths. India has entered into this phase.

(d) **Fourth stage:** In the fourth stage both birth and death rates are low and the resultant population is stationary. Hence this stage is also known as *low stationary stage.* This stage is seen in industrialized countries where a demographic transition has taken place from a high birth and death rates to a low birth and death rates. Austria attained a zero population growth during 1980-85.

(e) **Fifth stage:** This stage is characterized by fall in population hence it is also known as *declining stage*. Birth rate is lower than the death rate. Hungary and Germany are experiencing this stage.

Thus the demographic cycle is based on a **population balance equation**:

Population = Births – Deaths

The equation is useful at any time and at any stage in the demographic cycle. Using the equation given above all the five stages in the demographic cycle can be summarized in Table 3.2 as follows:

Table 3.2. Different stages in the demographic cycle

Stage	Birth rate	Death rate	Population
First stage (High stationary)	High	High	Stationary
Second stage (Early expanding)	No change	Decline	Increase
Third stage (Late expanding)	Decline	Further decline	Slight increase
Fourth stage (Low stationary)	Low	Low	Almost stationary
Fifth stage (Declining)	Lower	Low	Decrease

FERTILITY

Fertility means actual bearing of children. A woman's fertile age ranges between 15 to 45 years i.e. the reproductive period is of 30 years. During this period a woman is constantly exposed to the risk of pregnancy and may give birth to a maximum of 15 children. According to statistics, on an average a woman gives birth to six or seven children provided her married life is not interrupted. In 1985 the **Total Fertility Rates** (TFR) were minimum (1.5) in Switzerland, intermediate (4.5) in India and maximum (7.8) in Kenya. TFR gives an indication of total number of children borne by a woman during her reproductive age, 15 to 45 years. Such differences in TFR or fertility are due to several factors, important factors for India being low age at marriage, universality of marriage, low level of literacy, poor standard of living, less popularity of family planning programs, limited use of contraceptives and traditional ways of living.

High fertility rate in India can be brought down through various measures, which are related to the following factors:

(a) **Age at marriage:** Early marriage was a custom in India and child marriages are still solemnized. Prior to 1951 the average age at marriage of woman was 13 years, in 1961 it was 16.3 years and in 1981 it became 18.6 years. Age at marriage is the age at which a female marries and enters the reproductive life. It has a direct impact on the fertility. It can be easily expected that a female marrying before 18 years of age can give birth to a greater number of children than if she was married at the age of 20 years. But the average age at marriage of both men and women in India is increasing. This can bring down fertility and help in controlling the population.

(b) **Duration of married life:** It has been estimated that 50 to 55% births occur within 5 to 15 years of married life while 10 to 25% births occur within 1 to 5 years. These figures indicate that if the family planning efforts are focused within first few years of married life, the number of births can be easily controlled.

(c) **Spacing of children:** Fertility rates can be brought down by proper spacing of the children. Greater is the gap between the births of the children lower is the fertility rate. Postponement of all births just by one year will reduce fertility rate tremendously.

(d) **Education:** It is well established that the fertility rates are low in case of educated people. Thus educational status of people is inversely related to the fertility rates. This is the reason for high fertility rates in illiterate than literate people and similarly high fertility rates in rural population than in urban population where more people are educated. Educated people are definitely aware about the family welfare and hence the importance of a small family and less number of children.

(e) **Economic status:** Economic status also plays an important role in fertility. Thus fertility is lower in population with higher economic status. Improving economic status of the people is considered to be an effective method of controlling fertility i.e. population growth.

(f) **Caste and religion:** Caste and religion also play an important role in fertility. Fertility rates are higher in Muslims as compared to Hindus. Fertility rates are lower in higher castes amongst Hindus as compared to lower castes.

(g) **Nutrition:** Nutrition has an indirect effect on fertility. Poorly fed societies exhibit high fertility rates whereas fed societies show lower fertility rates.

(h) **Family planning:** Family planning programs and their effective implementation are important in fertility reduction. These are more important in developing countries like India. Family planning programs are economical and have long term beneficial effect.

(i) **Other factors:** These factors are related to physical, biological, social and cultural aspects like health status of people, place of women and children in society, housing and health conditions, sanitation, hygiene, industrialization, medical facilities etc.

FAMILY PLANNING

Pharmacists are members of healthcare team. They are aware of the dangers of population and its explosion. They can realize the need of population control and the importance of family planning. Population control is the responsibility of a community but family planning is the responsibility of individual couples. Family planning is a way of life adopted by the married couples to promote the health and welfare of their families. Family planning refers to practices that help individuals to attain the following objectives.

A. Objectives

1. To avoid unwanted births and bring about wanted births.
2. To regulate the spacing between children.
3. To control the time at which births occur in relation to the age of parents.
4. To determine the number of children in the family.

According to WHO family planning is a way of thinking and living that is adopted voluntarily, upon the basis of knowledge, attitudes and responsive decisions by individuals and couples, in order to promote the health and welfare of the family group and thus contributes effectively to the social development of a country.

Family planning is a basic human right and all couples have a right to decide and plan the numbers and spacing of their children. Family planning and birth control are not synonymous although birth control is the most important component of family planning. Unfortunately the concept of family planning is not properly understood by many people. Some people associate it with sterility while others equate it with birth control. Both are misconceptions. Family planning is based on *welfare concept* and hence it has been rightly renamed as family welfare program. This point would be clear when we examine the scope of family planning.

B. Scope

Family planning has wide scope and includes the following activities:

1. Proper spacing and limitation of births.
2. Investigation and advice on sterility.
3. Education for parenthood.
4. Sex education.
5. Screening of the reproductive system for pathological conditions e.g. cervical cancer.
6. Genetic counseling.
7. Pre-marital consultations and examinations.
8. Carrying out pregnancy tests.
9. Marriage counseling.
10. Preparation of the couples for the arrival of their first child.
11. Providing services for the unmarried mothers.
12. Home science including home economics and nutrition.
13. Care of unmarried mothers and adoption services.

By understanding themselves and making the public understand the scope of family planning, pharmacists can do a great job, particularly in rural areas.

Only a couple can decide about the size of their family they would like to have. This includes the *number* of children as well as *spacing* between the children. Married couples can avoid unwanted pregnancies and regulate the proper spacing by adopting family planning measures. Contraception is only one of these measures.

Birth control is an umbrella term for several techniques and methods used to prevent fertilization or to interrupt pregnancy at various stages. Birth control techniques and methods include (a) *contraception* (the prevention of fertilization), (b) *contragestion* (the prevention of the implantation of the blastocyst), and (c) *abortion* (the removal or expulsion of a fetus or embryo from the uterus). Contraception includes barrier methods, such as condoms or diaphragm, hormonal contraception, also known as oral contraception, and injectable contraceptives. Contragestives, also known as post-coital birth control, include intrauterine devices (IUDs) and what is known as the emergency contraceptive.

CONTRACEPTION METHODS

Contraception methods are used to avoid unwanted pregnancies resulting from coitus (sexual intercourse). They are also used as fertility regulating methods. Contraceptive methods can be classified as shown in Figure 3.1.

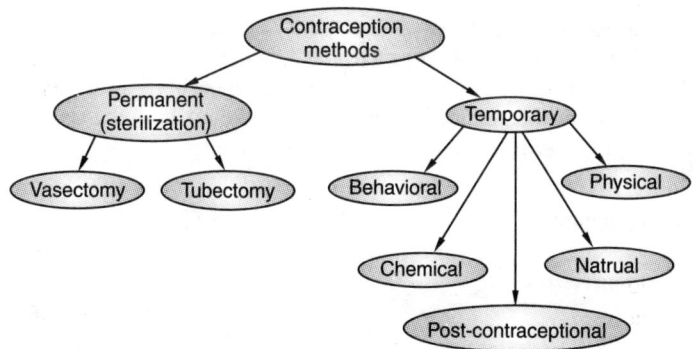

Fig. 3.1. Different methods of contraception.

An *ideal contraceptive* should be safe, effective, acceptable to both the partners, reversible, cheap, easily available and easy to use, independent of coitus, long lasting, free from side effects and should not require medical supervision. Thus there is no ideal contraceptive available yet contraception methods are widely used today. We are passing through an age of contraceptive revolution.

Each of the contraceptive methods or device has its own advantages and disadvantages and adoption of a particular method is purely a matter of individual couple's preference.

A. Temporary Methods of Contraception

(a) Behavioral Methods

These methods are simplest and their success depends on how the two partners to coitus behave.

(i) Abstinence

This is the most effective contraceptive method but not practical. It means that one should withhold from sex act which is probably unnatural and may lead to temperamental changes and even nervous breakdown.

(ii) Coitus interruptus

This method is based on interruption during coitus. During the coitus the male partner withdraws penis from female passage just before ejaculation and discharges outside. The deposition of the semen into the vagina is prevented. Thus coitus interruptus is a voluntary method and does not involve cost or appliance. However, some couples find it difficult in practice. The failure rate of this method may be as high as 18 and it is usually due to mistake in timing of withdrawal. Secondly, the pre-coital secretion of male may contain sperms and even a drop of semen is sufficient to cause pregnancy.

(iii) Rhythm method

It is also called as 'safe period' or 'calendar' method (Fig. 3.2). It was first described in 1930. Coitus is performed 7 to 8 days *before* and *after* menstrual flow. The method is based on the fact that ovulation occurs from 12 to 16 days before the onset of menstruation. The failure of the method is usually due to wrong calculation and irregular menstrual cycle in a woman.

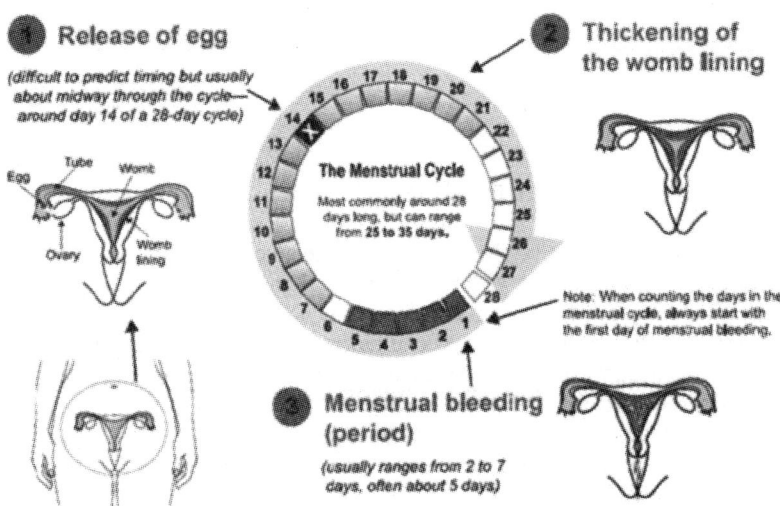

Fig. 3.2. Rhythm (Calendar) method.

Thus although behavioral methods are simple yet depend upon the will power of individual and cooperation of the partners. Programmed sex i.e. compulsory abstinence from sexual intercourse for nearly one half of every month seems to be safe and voluntary method of contraception.

(b) Physical Methods

(i) Male Condom

Condom and sheaths meet the requirement of an ideal contraceptive. Condom is popular in India. Most outstanding advantage of condom is that it protects both the partners from sexually transmitted diseases including AIDS. It is made from latex. The condom is applied on the erect penis before intercourse, air removed from the teat, and withdrawn from the vagina carefully after intercourse to avoid spilling of semen in the vagina (Fig. 3.3).

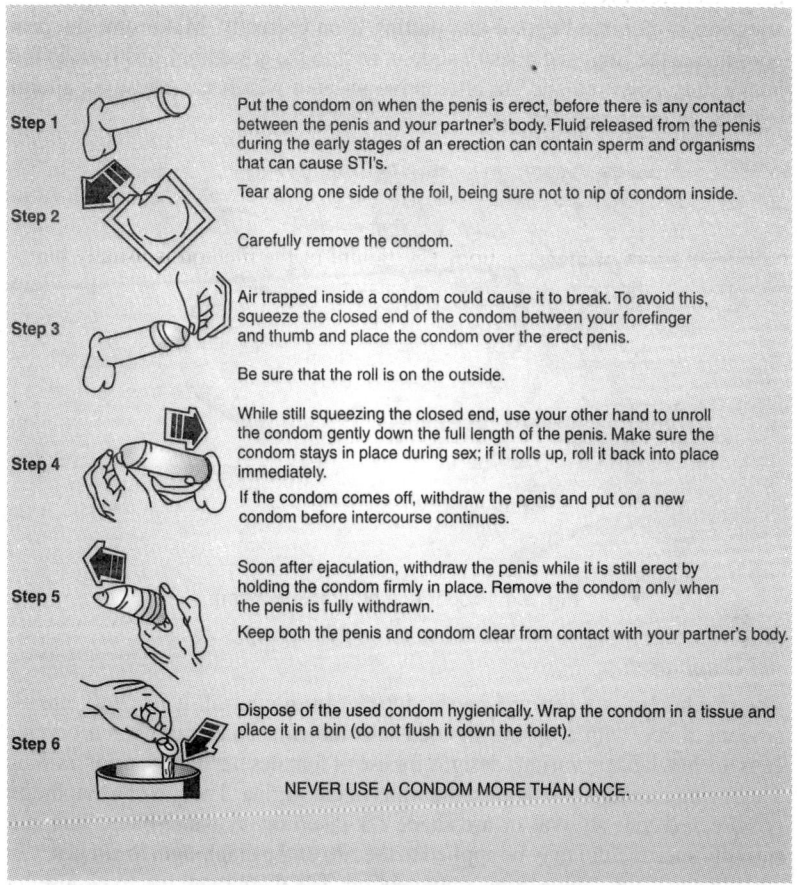

Step 1 Put the condom on when the penis is erect, before there is any contact between the penis and your partner's body. Fluid released from the penis during the early stages of an erection can contain sperm and organisms that can cause STI's.

Step 2 Tear along one side of the foil, being sure not to nip of condom inside.

Carefully remove the condom.

Step 3 Air trapped inside a condom could cause it to break. To avoid this, squeeze the closed end of the condom between your forefinger and thumb and place the condom over the erect penis.

Be sure that the roll is on the outside.

Step 4 While still squeezing the closed end, use your other hand to unroll the condom gently down the full length of the penis. Make sure the condom stays in place during sex; if it rolls up, roll it back into place immediately.

If the condom comes off, withdraw the penis and put on a new condom before intercourse continues.

Step 5 Soon after ejaculation, withdraw the penis while it is still erect by holding the condom firmly in place. Remove the condom only when the penis is fully withdrawn.

Keep both the penis and condom clear from contact with your partner's body.

Step 6 Dispose of the used condom hygienically. Wrap the condom in a tissue and place it in a bin (do not flush it down the toilet).

NEVER USE A CONDOM MORE THAN ONCE.

Fig. 3.3. Proper use of male condom (Nirodh).

Nirodh is a Sanskrit word meaning prevention. Three types of condoms are made available by the Government of India at highly subsidized cost (i) Dry-Nirodh, (ii) a lubricated Deluxe Nirodh, and (iii) a thinner variety, the Super Deluxe Nirodh. These condoms are distributed free of cost in Primary Health Centres (PHC), Community Health Centres (CHC), and District Hospitals. Various other types of condoms are also available in the market like *Kohinoor, Moods dotted condom, Durex, Masti, Climax* etc.

(ii) Female Condom

The female condom is designed to be worn by women during penetration. The female condom has a small, flexible ring on the closed end, designed to cover the cervix, and a larger ring that remains on the outside of the receiver's body (Fig. 3.4). Female condoms don't sheath the penis tightly, so a little more attention is required beyond just putting it on correctly. Make sure the penis goes inside the ring, and doesn't slide in next to the condom. Construction is of heavy duty polyurethane, an alternative to latex which can cause an allergic reaction in some people.

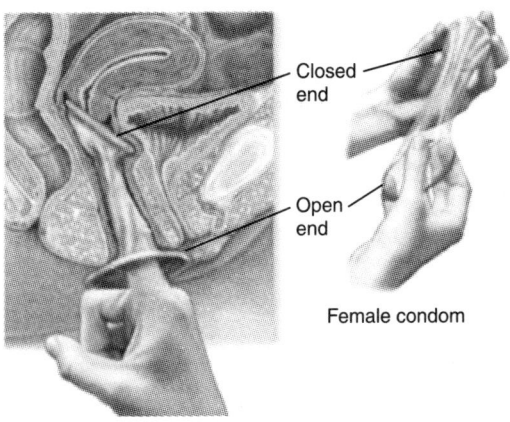

Female condom

Fig. 3.4. Proper use of female condom.

(iii) Diaphragm

The diaphragm is a cervical barrier type of birth control. It is a soft latex or silicone dome with a spring molded into the rim. Diaphragms and cervical caps are available in various designs for use of females but require prior training. The spring creates a seal against the walls of the vagina. The rim of a diaphragm is squeezed into an oval or arc shape for insertion. A water-based lubricant (usually spermicide) may be applied to the rim of the diaphragm to aid insertion and enhances the safety from contraception. The diaphragm has to be inserted before sexual intercourse and must remain in place for at least 6 hours after intercourse. Upon removal, a diaphragm should be cleansed with warm mild soapy water before storage. The diaphragm must be removed for cleaning at least once every 24 hours and can be re-inserted immediately.

Oil-based products should not be used with latex diaphragms. Lubricants or vaginal medications that contain oil will cause the latex to rapidly degrade and greatly increase the chances of breaking or tearing of the diaphragm. Natural latex rubber will degrade over time. Depending on usage and storage conditions, a latex diaphragm should be replaced every one to three years. Silicone diaphragms may last much longer – up to ten years.

A correctly fitted diaphragm will cover the cervix and rest snugly against the "glen" of the Pelvis bone. The spring in the rim of the diaphragm forms a seal against the vaginal walls. The diaphragm covers the cervix, and physically prevents sperm from entering the uterus.

Diaphragms are available in diameters of 50 mm to 105 mm (about 2–4 inches). They are available in two different materials: latex and silicone. The SILCS diaphragm is made of silicone, while Duet disposable diaphragm is made of dipped polyurethane, pre-filled with BufferGel, a spermicide. Diaphragms are also available with different types of springs in the rim. Common varieties of diaphragm include cervical cap, vault cap and the vimule cap (Fig. 3.5). Diaphragms were very popular before oral contraceptives came in practice.

Table 3.3. Different types of diaphragm

Types of Diaphragm	Features	Examples
Arcing spring	It folds into an arc shape when the sides are compressed. This is the strongest type of rim available in a diaphragm. Arcing spring diaphragms may be easier to insert correctly than other spring types.	Ortho All-Flex and Milex Wide-Seal Arcing
Coil spring	It flattens into an oval shape when the sides are compressed. This rim is not as strong as the arcing spring.	Ortho Coil, Milex Wide-Seal Omniflex, and Semina
Flat spring	It is much like a coil spring, but thinner. These may also be inserted with the help of an introducer.	Ortho White

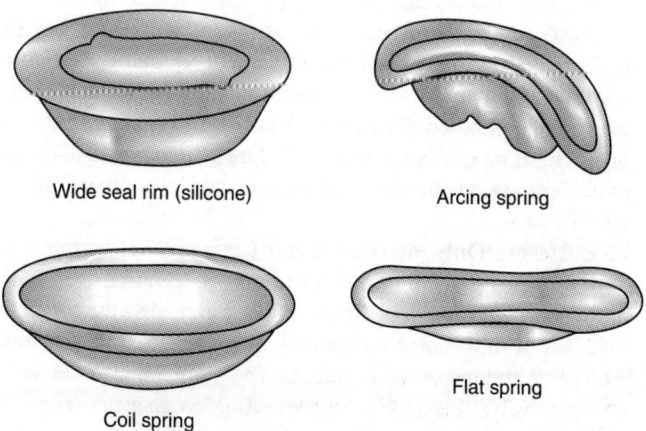

Wide seal rim (silicone)　　　　　Arcing spring

Coil spring　　　　　Flat spring

Fig. 3.5. Common varieties of diaphragm.

(iv) Vaginal sponge

It is a small polyurethane foam sponge saturated with spermicides. It is lesser effective than diaphragm and not used in India.

(c) Chemical Methods

In conventional methods a spermicide is incorporated in the base and the product is used as (i) foam tablets or foam aerosols, (ii) creams, jellies and pastes, (iii) suppositories, and (iv) soluble films. However these methods of contraception are not really safe and reliable.

(i) Hormonal Contraceptives

Hormonal contraceptives are most popular all over the world including India. They are almost cent per cent effective in preventing pregnancy and ensuring spacing between child births. Steroidal hormones used as contraceptives include synthetic estrogens e.g. ethinylestradiol and mestranol, and synthetic progestogens: (i) pregnanes e.g. megestrol and medroxy-progesterone acetate; (ii) estrogens e.g. norethisterone, lynesterol and norethysterone acetate; and (iii) gonanes e.g. levonorgesterol. Hormonal contraceptives are used in two forms (a) Oral pills, and (b) Depot formulations.

(a) **Oral pills**

    (i) **Combined Pills:** It contains combination hormones, 30 to 35 mcg of a synthetic estrogen and 0.5 to 1 mg of a progestogen. It prevents the release of the ovum from the ovary by blocking the pituitary secretion of gonadotrophin, which is necessary for the occurrence of ovulation. The pill is given orally for 21 consecutive days beginning on the fifth day of the menstrual period. The pill must be taken everyday at a fixed time at night before going to bed. It might be followed by one iron tablet. **Mala-N** (containing 1 mg of norethisterone acetate and 0.03 mg of ethinylestradiol) and **Mala-D** (containing 0.5 mg of D-norgestrel and 0.03 mg of ethinylestradiol) are the examples of low dose pills both made available by the Government of India. Post-coital (after unprotected intercourse) contraception can also be achieved through the use of combined pill within 48 hours. In situation like unprotected intercourse, rape or contraception failure a double dose of the combined pills (2 pills) is given immediately, followed by another 2 pills 12 hours later.

    (ii) **Progesterone Only Pill (POP):** POP ('*minipill*' or '*micropill*') contains only progestogen; either norethisterone or levonorgesterol, and given in small doses throughout the cycle. The pill renders the cervical mucous thick and scanty, which inhibits the sperm penetration. The transport of the sperm and the ovum to the uterine cavity are also delayed. POP is also nearly 100% effective in preventing pregnancy. Failure occurs if the pill is not taken regularly.

i-pill is an emergency contraceptive pill. It contains levonorgestrel – a progestogen, which helps prevent the implantation of the egg in the uterus and avoids the beginning of pregnancy. *i-pill* can work in any of the three different ways:

• It may stop an egg being released from the ovary.
• If an egg has been released, it may prevent the sperm from fertilizing it.
• If the egg is already fertilized, it may prevent it from attaching itself to the lining of the womb.

A single dose of *i-pill* provides a safe and easy way to prevent an unintended pregnancy after unprotected sex or contraceptive failure.

(iii) **Centchroman Tablets:** A tablet recently introduced in India is *Saheli*, which contains centchroman. Centchroman is a non-steroidal birth control tablet for use by woman. Initially it should be taken twice a week for first three months and then once a week. It is free from the typical side-effects of hormonal contraceptives. It is a safe, oral contraceptive. Contraceptive action is reversible within six months. Nursing mothers should not use *Saheli* during the first six months of the post-natal period.

Oral contraceptive pills are widely used in western countries and they are also becoming popular in India. They are highly effective as contraceptive without any effect on sexual activity.

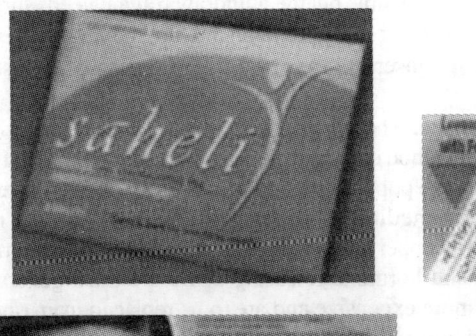
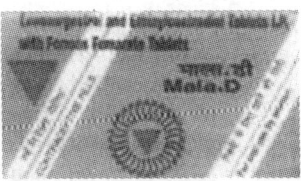
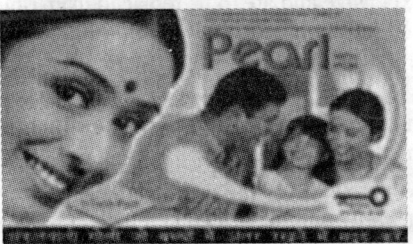
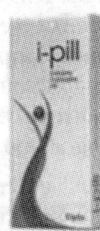

Fig. 3.6. Commonly used oral pills.

(b) **Depot Formulations:** As against oral pills which are to be taken daily, *single* administration of depot preparations is sufficient for several months or years. They are highly effective, reversible, long acting, and estrogen free. They can be injected into the body (injectable contraceptives), implanted beneath the skin (implants) or worn in the vagina (vaginal rings).

1. **Injectable contraceptives**

   (i) **DMPA:** One intramuscular injection (150 mg) of DMPA (Depot-Medroxy Progesterone Acetate or Depot-provera) is sufficient for ninety days. DMPA suppresses ovulation. It is safe, effective and acceptable contraceptive, which does not affect lactation. It is suitable for spacing pregnancies. Its disadvantages include weight increase, irregular menstrual and prolonged infertility after its use. Depot provera is the most controversial contraceptive in India.

   (ii) **Norethisterone enantate (NET-EN):** It is given intramuscularly in a dose of 60 mg every 60 days. It is less popular than DMPA. It also inhibits ovulation like DMPA. The initial injection of both DMPA and NET-EN (deep intramuscular) should be given during the first five days of menstrual period. Both contraceptives are reversible.

2. **Subdermal implants:** These are implanted subdermally, beneath the skin of the forearm or upper arm by surgical procedure for long term contraception extending over 5 years. *Norplant* is a capsule containing levonorgrsterol. *Norplant R-2* also contain levonorgesterol but in the form of rods. On withdrawal of the implant pregnancy occurs as usual hence contraception is reversible but the withdrawal again needs surgical procedure. Disadvantages of these implants include (i) requirement of surgical procedure for insertion, and (ii) irregularities of menstrual bleeding.

   (i) **Intrauterine devices:** The intrauterine device (IUD) is the world's most widely used method of reversible birth control for women. IUDs have recently become popular as contraceptive. These may be either medicated or non-medicated. First generation IUDs are non-medicated or inert, copper IUDs are considered as second generation IUDs (Fig. 3.7) and hormone releasing IUDs are third generation IUDs. IUDs are more expensive and are to be replaced from time to time but they are quite effective.

   (ii) **Lippes loop:** It is a double-S shaped plastic loop inserted into uterine cavity through cervix with the help of a plastic cylinder. It has now been replaced by Copper T. Loop was included in the National Family Programme of Government of India in 1961.

   Second generation IUDs are based on the use of copper due to its strong anti-fertility effect. Copper devices are effective, well tolerated, easier to fit (Fig. 3.8) and have low incident of side effects e.g. pain and bleeding. Commonly used devices include Copper-7, Copper T-220 C,

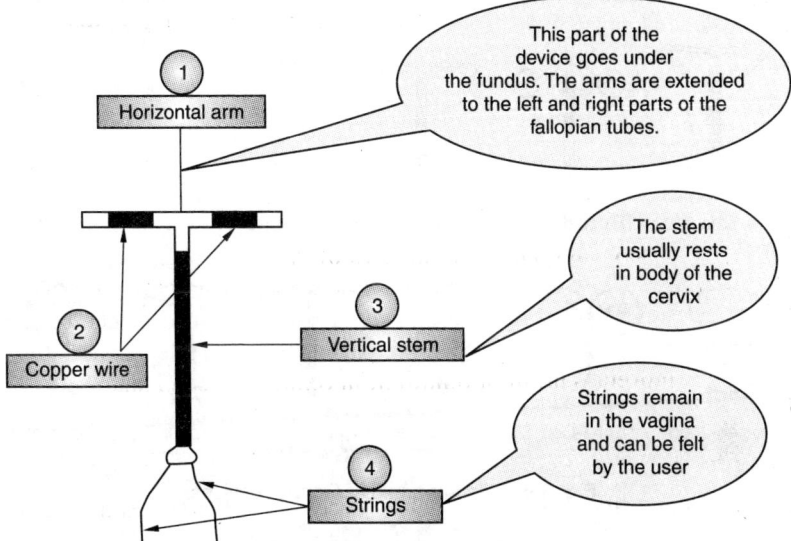

Fig. 3.7. Copper-T.

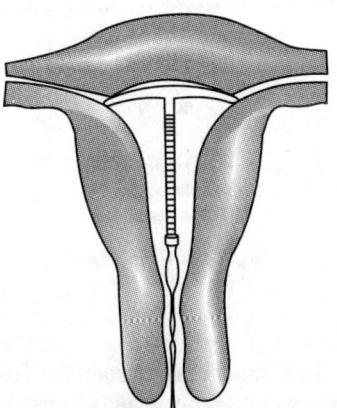

Fig. 3.8. Position of IUD in uterus.

T Cu-380 A or AG, Nova T and Multi-load devices (ML-Cu and ML-Cu-375) (Fig. 3.9). Number 7 and letter T in the names refer to the shape while other numbers indicate the surface area in sq. mm of the copper in the device. T Cu-380 Ag has a silver core over which copper wire is wrapped. Copper devices are very popular in India.

Third generation IUDs are based on the use of a hormone e.g. progesterone or levonorgesterol as a contraceptive agent. Progestasert (Fig. 3.10) releases 65 mcg/ day of progesterone for a period of 1 year.

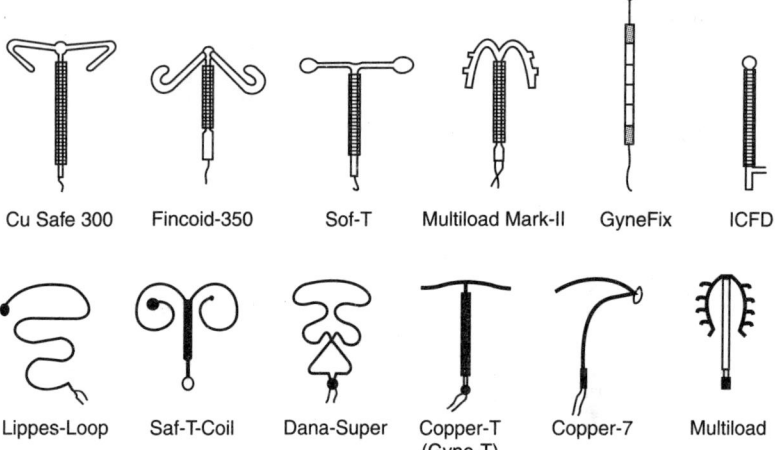

Cu Safe 300   Fincoid-350   Sof-T   Multiload Mark-II   GyneFix   ICFD

Lippes-Loop   Saf-T-Coil   Dana-Super   Copper-T (Gyne-T)   Copper-7   Multiload

Fig. 3.9. Different types of Copper devices.

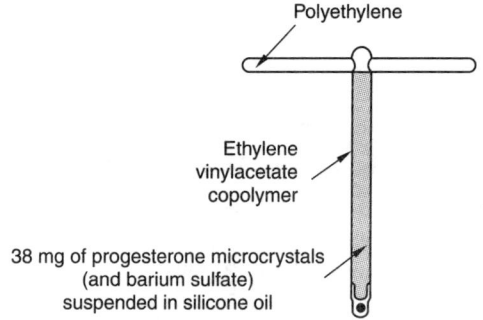

Polyethylene

Ethylene vinylacetate copolymer

38 mg of progesterone microcrystals (and barium sulfate) suspended in silicone oil

Fig. 3.10. Progestasert.

(d) Natural Methods

Pregnancy can be avoided if the couples abstain from sexual intercourse during the fertile period of the menstrual cycle and obviously the woman should be able to ascertain when the fertile period begins. Thus in the natural family planning methods the women employ self recognition of certain physiological signs and symptoms associated with ovulation. There is no need to use any drugs or contraceptives devices. There are three recognized natural family planning methods.

(i) Basal Body Temperature (BBT) method

At the time of ovulation the production of progesterone increases and this results in the rise of BBT by 0.3 to 0.5°C. The body temperature does not rise if ovulation does not occur. The temperature should be measured in the morning before getting out of bed. Pregnancy does not occur if intercourse is restricted to the post-ovulatory infertile period starting 3 days after the ovulatory temperature rise and continuing upto the beginning of menstruation. Very few couples use this method because abstinence is necessary for the entire pre-ovulatory period.

(ii) Billing's method

It is also known as cervical mucous method or ovulation method. The woman should be able to distinguish between different types of mucus. The quantity and characteristic of mucus can be observed by the woman by using a tissue paper to wipe the inside of the vagina. During the time of ovulation the cervical mucus becomes watery clear like raw egg white, smooth, slippery and profuse. After ovulation the mucus becomes thicker and lesser in quantity due to the production of progesterone. Billing's method is not much practiced in India.

(iii) Symptothermic method

It is more effective than the Billing's method and is based on identifying the fertile period by combined techniques of BBT, cervical mucus and calendar method. It serves as a double check if the woman is unable to interpret clearly one sign.

Natural family planning methods can be practiced by those who can impose self discipline and understand sex. These methods are not of much importance in developing countries.

(e) Post-contraception Methods

The methods used *after* the pregnancy has occurred are called post-contraceptional methods.

(i) Abortion

It means termination of pregnancy before the foetus becomes viable. The Medical Termination of Pregnancy Act 1971 states (i) the conditions under which a pregnancy can be terminated, (ii) the persons who can perform such termination, and (iii) the places where such termination can be performed (for details please refer A Textbook of Forensic Pharmacy by N. K. Jain; Vallabh Prakashan, Delhi)

(ii) Menstrual regulation

This is a relatively simple method of birth control. Uterine contents are aspirated 6 to 14 days of a missing period.

(iii) Menstrual induction

In this method normal progesterone-prostaglandin balance is disturbed by intrauterine application of 1 to 5 mg solution of prostaglandin F2. The uterus responds with a sustained contraception lasting about 7 minutes. This is followed by cyclic contraction continuing for 3 to 4 hours. The bleeding starts and continues for 7 to 8 days.

B. Permanent Methods of Contraception

Sterilization

It means the operative techniques called *vasectomy* in males and *tubectomy* in females. Vasectomy is relatively quick. Both the vas deferens are cut and tied as shown in (Fig. 3.11) and therefore sperms cannot enter the uterus. For females the technique of laparoscopic sterilization (Fig. 3.12) has been developed. A laparoscope is used to look into the abdominal cavity; both the fallopian tubes are cut and tied (tubal ligation). The tubal ligation is performed 4 to 7 days after delivery and the operation takes only 2 to 3 minutes. Sterilization is very effective and permanently safe method. It is ideal for those couples having two or more children. The Government is encouraging permanent methods by providing monetary incentives for sterilization and IUDs. Central and State Governments offer special incentives to their employees for adopting permanent methods of family planning.

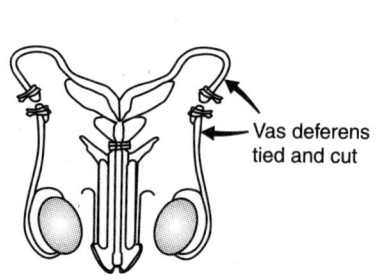

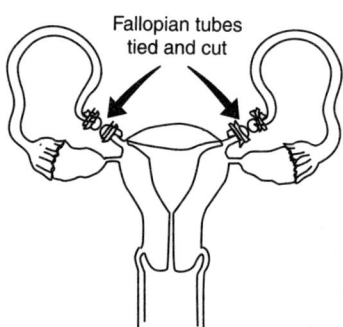

Fallopian tubes tied and cut

Vas deferens tied and cut

Fig. 3.11. Vasectomy.

Fig. 3.12. Tubectomy.

RECOMMENDED FAMILY PLANNING METHODS

The following methods of contraception and sterilization are usually recommended.

Newly married couples	Condom (Nirodh)
For couple having one child	Loops or Oral Pill (for spacing)
After second child	Sterilization

Spacing method is becoming more popular than sterilization programme but sterilization is the best method for those couples having larger families.

POPULATION PROBLEMS OF INDIA

India is one of the countries facing population problems. India is supporting 16% of the world's population with only 2% of the world's land area. Next to China, India is the world's second most populous country. Area-wise India is only two-fifths the size of USA but population wise India is more than triple of

Table 3.4. Comparison of Family Planning Methods

Method	Mode of action	Appropriateness	Non-appropriateness	Comments
Female Sterilization (Tubectomy)	Blocking of the fallopian tubes, so that sperm and egg cannot meet.	For women with a complete family.	When there is doubt whether more children will be wanted later, also not immediately after delivery.	Can be reversed, but with difficulty and uncertain success.
Male Sterilization (Vasectomy)	Blocking the vas deferens, so that no sperm cells are ejaculated.	For men with a complete family.	When there is doubt whether more children will be wanted later.	Semen test has to show that there are no sperm cells, before other methods of contraception can be stopped. Can be reversed, but with difficulty and uncertain success.
Implant	One or two small plastic rods, under the skin in the upper arm, release progestagen, which makes the mucus of the cervix impenetrable to sperm cells, and in most women also stops ovulation.	For women who want 2–3 years of contraception, without having to think about it.	When some irregular bleeding is unacceptable.	Works for 3–5 years, needs to be removed if pregnancy is desired.
Injection	Injection with progestagen, which makes the mucus of the cervix impenetrable to sperm cells and also stops ovulation in most women.	For women who want 12 weeks of contraception, without having to think about it.	When some irregular bleeding is unacceptable.	Works for 12 weeks, cannot be removed after injection, needs to be repeated if continued contraception is needed.

(Contd.)

Method	Mode of action	Appropriateness	Non-appropriateness	Comments
Vaginal ring	Releases an estrogen and a progestagen, which stop ovulation.	For women who only want to think twice per month about contraception.	For smokers, or for women with thrombosis in their history.	Works for 3 weeks when in the vagina, then has to be replaced after a stop week.
Patch	Releases an estrogen and a progestagen, which stop ovulation.	For women who only want to think about contraception once a week.	For smokers, or for women with thrombosis in their history.	Not well suited in humid climates, can be visible.
Combined oral contraceptive pill	Contains an estrogen and a progestagen, which stop ovulation.	For women who want to take a pill daily.	For smokers, for women with thrombosis in their history, for women who tend to forget daily pill intake.	—
Progestagen only pill (POP), or estrogen free pill	Contains a progestagen, which makes the mucus of the cervix impenetrable to sperm cells and in a number of women also blocks ovulation.	For women who do not want or cannot take estrogen.	For women who tend to forget daily pill intake.	Most progestagen only pills must not be taken more than 3 hours late, but some can be taken up to 12 hours late.
Intrauterine device (IUD) with hormone	Makes mucus of the cervix impenetrable to sperm and prevents implantation of an egg.	For women who only want to think about contraception once in 5 years.	For women at risk for sexually transmitted disease.	Women need to check regularly whether it is still in place. IUD needs to be replaced after 5 years.
IUD plain	Prevents implantation of an egg.	For women who do not want to think about contraception for a number of years.	For women with heavy menstruation, or for women at risk for sexually transmitted disease.	Women need to check regularly whether it is still in place.

(*Contd.*)

Method	Mode of action	Appropriateness	Non-appropriateness	Comments
Male condom	Prevents sperm entering the vagina.	For men whose partner cannot or does not want to take contraceptives, for men with multiple partners, for men with infrequent intercourse.	—	Provides some protection against sexually transmitted diseases and AIDS.
Female condom	Prevents sperm entering the vagina.	For women who cannot or do not want to use other contraceptives, who have multiple partners or infrequent intercourse.	—	Provides some protection against sexually transmitted diseases and AIDS.
Diaphragm	Prevents sperm from entering the uterus.	For women who cannot or do not want to use other contraceptives, who have multiple partners or infrequent intercourse.	For women who are not familiar with their vagina.	Has to be used with a spermicide.

USA. India's population is increasing at the rate of 16 million per year, growth rate is 2.2%. Already containing 17.5% of the world's population, India is projected to be the world's most populous country by 2025, surpassing China, its population reaching 1.6 billion by 2050. The population trend in India during 20th century is indicated in Table 3.5.

Table 3.5. Population of India in 20th century

Census year	Total population (Millions)
1901	238.4
1911	252.1
1921	251.3
1931	279.0
1941	318.7
1951	361.1
1961	439.2
1971	548.2
1981	683.3
1991	846.4
2001	1028.7
2011	1210.2

Six States i.e. Uttar Pradesh, Bihar, Maharashtra, West Bengal, Andhra Pradesh and Madhya Pradesh account for nearly 60% of India's population. The statistics of census 2011 are sufficient to project the alarming population problem of India. Inspite of the tremendous progress made by the country the benefits are not reaching the public due to increasing population. To some extent this rising population has been checked due to government's policies and family welfare programmes but life expectancy has also increased due to better health facilities and advances in medical sciences. Poverty and illiteracy are root causes of population problem in India. Effective implementation of National Health Policy, popularizing voluntary family planning specially in rural areas; and making the people, particularly below the poverty line, aware of the hazards of the population explosion and need for 2 children family norm are some of the measures that can solve the population problem of India.

First-Aid

INTRODUCTION

First-aid is the immediate, temporary emergency aid given by a lay man to a sufferer in case of medical emergency (accident or sudden illness). Early measures may be useful in saving life and ensuring a better and faster recovery. The avoidance of unnecessary movement and over-excitation of the victim often prevents further injury.

The duty of the first-aider is to render aid until the arrival of a physician. Once the medical practitioner takes the complete charge, the responsibility of the first-aider ceases. Proper first-aid may save the life of a patient and reduce his suffering. Everybody should take first-aid training because medical emergency may arise any where and at any time. But as pharmacists our responsibility is still greater because people expect much more from pharmacists and this is justified in view of their knowledge and training.

The generalized objectives of every first-aid training program are:

1. Prevention of accidents by means of safety campaigns and instruction in the fundamentals of first-aid, whenever possible.
2. Teaching the first-aider to determine the appropriate type and extent of injury so that patient suffers minimum harm when the assistance is rendered.
3. Teaching the first-aider to act quickly and efficiently in case of an emergency. A first-aider should know the do's and don'ts of the method of treatment.

AIMS OF FIRST-AID

The key aims of first-aid can be summarized in three key points:

1. Preserve life: The primary aim of all medical care, including first-aid, is to save lives.

2. Prevent further harm: It is also sometimes called *prevent the condition from worsening,* or *danger of further injury.* This covers both external factors, such as moving a patient away from any cause of harm, and applying first-aid techniques to prevent worsening of the condition, such as applying pressure to stop a bleed becoming dangerous.

3. Promote recovery: First-aid also involves trying to start the recovery process from the illness or injury, and in some cases might involve completing a treatment, such as in the case of applying a plaster to a small wound.

First-aid training also involves the prevention of initial injury and responder safety, and the treatment phases. Certain skills are considered essential to the provision of first-aid and are taught universally. Particularly the **ABCs** of first-aid, which focuses on critical life saving intervention that must be rendered before treatment of less serious injuries. ABC stands for *Airway, Breathing,* and *Circulation.* Attention must first be brought to the airway to ensure that it is clear. Obstruction (choking) is a life-threatening emergency. Following evaluation of the airway, a first-aid attendant would determine adequacy of breathing and provide rescue breathing, if necessary. Assessment of circulation is now not usually carried out for patients who are not breathing, with first-aiders now trained to go straight to chest compressions (and thus providing artificial circulation) but pulse checks may be done on less serious patients.

Some organizations add a fourth step of "**D**" for *Deadly bleeding* or *Defibrillation,* while others consider this as part of the *Circulation* step. Variations on techniques to evaluate and maintain the ABCs depend on the skill level of the first-aider. Once the ABCs are secured, first-aiders can begin additional treatments, as required.

ABCs of first-aid are also described as the **3Bs**: *Breathing, Bleeding,* and *Bones* or **4Bs**: *Breathing, Bleeding, Brain,* and *Bones.* While the ABCs and 3Bs are taught to be performed sequentially, certain conditions may require the consideration of two steps simultaneously. This includes the provision of both *artificial respiration* and *chest compression* to someone who is not breathing and has no pulse, and the consideration of cervical spine injuries when ensuring an open airway.

The most important **Rules of first-aid** in order of importance are:

1. Supply oxygen to the lungs.
2. Stop bleeding.
3. Prevent and treat shock.
4. Prevent further injury.
5. Call physician, hospital poison control center or rescue until transport vehicle to a medical facility is available.

EMERGENCY TREATMENT

(a) Shock

Shock is a serious condition present to some extent in every injury. It may prove fatal. Shock occurs when the circulation system fails to send blood to all parts of the body. With shock, blood flow or blood volume is too low to meet the body's needs. Areas of the body are deprived of oxygen. The result is damage to the limbs, lungs, heart, and brain. Loss of blood from any injury can cause shock. It can be characterized by depression of body functions, particularly the nervous system and circulation. There are many different forms of shocks with different apparent causes. Shock may be reversible or irreversible.

Symptoms

Symptoms of shocks are weakness, trembling, feeling restless, confusion, pale or blue-coloured lips, skin, and/or fingernails; cool and moist skin, rapid, shallow breathing, weak but fast pulse, nausea, vomiting, extreme thirst, dilated pupils in later stages, and sometimes unconsciousness.

Treatment

It is necessary to ascertain that the patient is suffering from shock. Whether on the ground or on bed, the patient should be placed in a reclining position with his or her feet higher than his or her head but do not raise the feet or move the legs if hip or leg bones are broken. In this condition, let the person lie flat. The body position should be adjusted according to the victim's injuries. If any external bleeding is observed then steps must be taken to stop it immediately. If the person vomits or has breathing trouble, raise him or her to a half-sitting position (if no head, back, or neck injury) or turn the person on his or her side to prevent choking.

Patient must be kept warm by placing a blanket, coat or even newspapers under as well as over the patient. In cold weather, hot water bottles can be used. Necessary steps should be taken to relieve pain by making the patient comfortable. If the injury is a fracture and medical aid is not immediately available then pain can be relieved by suitable splinting. Intense pain can also be relieved by medication such as morphine or other pain killers. If the patient is conscious he or she should be given as much fluid to drink as he or she can tolerate comfortably. Fluids containing sugar and salt are excellent e.g. orange juice, ginger ale or water with a teaspoonful of salt added. If the patient is unable to take fluids by mouth, a sugar or salt solution may be administered by rectum in the form of a retention enema. The solution may contain about a teaspoonful of sugar or salt in a glass of water and run very slowly into the rectum through a tube inserted about 6 inches.

(b) Electric shock

It includes the effects of the passage of electricity through the body. Fatality may result from shocks from 1 to 2 amperes and 500 to 1000 volts. Following conditions may arise during electric shock: it makes a person fall down, muscle contraction, seizures, dehydration, burns, fractures, clotting of blood, tissue death (narcosis) and respiratory/heart/kidney failure.

Treatment

For the treatment of electric shock, electric current should be shut off immediately and the victim pulled away. While releasing the victim don't touch wire, source of current or victim's body. Any metallic article should not be touched with bare hands. Rescuer should stand on a dry board or other non-conducting materials (such as dry rubber soles) and drag the patient from the contact with one hand that has been thickly insulated in some non-conducting materials such as rubber, dry clothes or several layers of paper; or making a loop of dry rope on a dry stick and by looping this over the victim's hand or foot. Soon after breaking the contact the victim should be brought in a semi-recumbent position. Upon recovery, such patients are likely to show hysterical outbursts and may attempt to run away, completely disoriented. If the patient becomes violent, he/she should be guarded against himself/herself.

Prevention

Some preventive measures to avoid electric shock are as follow:

1. Proper design, installation, maintenance of electric devices.
2. Educating the public regarding electrical devices.
3. Keep electrical gadgets out of children's reach.
4. Learn to respect electricity and electrical devices.

(c) Snake bite

Globally, thousands of people suffer from snake bites every year. Snake bites are very common in India, particularly in rural areas and a large number of deaths occur every year. Some common venomous snakes include Viper, Cobra, Rattle snake, Water moccasin, Coral snake, and Copper head. These deaths due to snake bite can be avoided if the victims get the first-aid.

Symptoms

The signs and symptoms of the snake bite are – fang marks, swelling/severe pain at the site, bloody discharge from wound, burning, diarrhoea, excessive sweating, blurred vision, numbness/tingling sensation, increased thirst, vomiting, fever, loss of muscle co-ordinations, convulsions, rapid pulse, and weakness/dizziness/fainting.

Treatment

Seek medical help as soon as possible. Meanwhile, wash the wound with soap/water and immobilize the affected area. Apply a firm bandage 2–4 inches above bite to prevent venom from spreading or apply a **tourniquet** (tourniquet is a compression device, which is used to cut off the flow of blood to a part of the body, most often an arm or leg tightly enough above the wound to check venous return circulation *but not to shut off circulation to the limb*). If necessary, keep moving tourniquet upwards as swelling extends. Open the holes made by the snake's fangs with a sharp knife or razor blade, which has been sterilized by passing it through a flame. If possible, cut across and length wise. The blood is allowed to run from the knife-cut. Alternately the wound can be sucked and expectorated. Any possible treatment for shock should also be given. The patient should be moved to a doctor as soon as possible. Pressure should be continued/maintained. It is safer to travel in snake infested area with emergency snake bite kit.

Prevention

Do not attempt to kill a snake. If you spot a snake, leave it alone. While hiking or in the woods, stay out of tall grass, Do not put your hand into pits/crevices during treks and keep caution while climbing rocks.

(d) Burns

Burns can be classified according to the nature of damage to the tissues e.g. first degree, second degree and third degree; corresponding, respectively to reddening of the skin, blistering of the skin and destruction of the skin or underlying parts. The danger to the body is proportionate to the extensiveness of the burn. A mild burn over a large area is more dangerous than a second degree burn of small size. All burns are painful. Shock is usually severe in burns over a large area.

Symptoms

Redness (first-degree burns), blistering (second-degree burns), charring of skin (third-degree burns).

Treatment

The concept of burn treatment has undergone radical change. Earlier it was believed that burn should be protected from water but today it is recommended that water be poured over the burn. This relieves the pain and prevents the damage to the affected area. The first-aid treatment of burns involves relief of pain and the treatment of shock. Doctor should be called immediately. Cold water may be applied to first- and second-degree burns. All burns should be covered with sterile, non-adherent dressings. Pains in mild burns of first degree may be relieved by the application of a burn ointment or a solution of baking soda. Second and third degree burns are best treated by applying sterile gauge saturated with a slightly warm baking soda solution. Solutions can be prepared by adding 2 to 3 teaspoonfuls of baking soda to 1 liter of previously boiled water. A primary non-adherent gauge dressing can be held in place by a lightly applied bandage or by covering it with a large cloth.

Burns caused by chemicals should be washed with large quantity of water; vinegar may be added to the water for alkali burns, and sodium bicarbonate may be added to the water in case of acid burns and then treated as above. Burns due to strong acids should be washed with water followed by warm solutions of baking soda. Burns from strong alkalis should be washed with water, then dilute vinegar or boric acid solution is applied, followed by a burn ointment.

When the clothes catch fire, roll the person on the floor to extinguish the flames or envelope him in a coat, blanket, table cover etc, whichever is available at hand, and roll him from side to side. Any loose clothing should be cut away. Then follow the treatment as given above.

In case of sunburns apply Calamine Lotion, bland oil or a suitable first-aid ointment. In case of blistering don't open the blister. Apply a dressing of sterile gauge.

(e) Poisoning

Poisons are substances that cause injury, illness or death. These events are caused by a chemical activity in the cells. Poisons can be injected, inhaled or swallowed. Poisoning should be suspected if a person is sick for unknown reason. Poor ventilation can aggravate inhalation poisoning. First-aid is critical in saving the life of victims. The causes of poisoning may be medications, drug overdose, occupational exposure, cleaning detergents/paints, carbon mono oxide gas from furnace, insecticides, certain cosmetics, certain household plants, animals, and food poisoning (Botulism).

Symptoms

Blue lips, skin rashes, difficulty in breathing, diarrhoea, vomiting/nausea, fever, headache, giddiness/drowsiness, double vision, abdominal/chest pain, palpitations/irritability, loss of appetite, loss of bladder control, numbness, muscle twitching, seizures, weakness, pupils contracted to pin-point size from morphine or narcotics, and loss of consciousness.

Treatment

The golden rule for the first-aid treatment of poisoning is to remove the poison from contact with the patient and to obtain definite medical care at the earliest possible moment. A universal anti-dote contains Ipecac and activated charcoal; the latter absorbs the poison and the former causes it to be expelled. Pharmacist should not perform or recommend treatment for poisoning except for sample first-aid measure given below:

1. **Swallowed Poisons:** A physician should be called immediately and in the meantime first-aid treatment rendered. Try and identify the poison if possible. Check for signs like burns around mouth, breathing difficulty or vomiting. In case of convulsions, protect the person from self injury. If possible, patient should drink one or two glasses of water to dilute the poison. The patient should be made to vomit by giving one ounce of Syrup of Ipecac with a cup of water. If vomiting does not occur in 20 minutes, then the dose is repeated. If Ipecac Syrup is not available, then vomiting may be induced by tickling back of throat with spoon handle or other blunt object, after giving water. Vomiting is not recommended in following conditions: *(i)* when the patient is unconscious or having fits, or *(ii)* when the patient has swallowed a poison containing kerosene or other gasoline or other petroleum distillate. Position the victim on the left till medical help arrives.

2. **Inhaled Poisons:** These include fuel gases, auto exhaust, and dense smoke from fire or fumes of poisonous chemicals. Take precaution before you attempt to rescue others. Hold a wet cloth to cover your nose and mouth. Open all the doors and windows. Take deep breaths before you begin the rescue. Patient should be moved into fresh air and his clothes loosened. Avoid lighting a match. If the patient vomits, take steps to prevent choking. Check the patient's breathing. If patient is not breathing properly, he/she should be given artificial respiration promptly till he/she starts breathing well or help arrives.

Steps to Avoid

1. Avoid giving an unconscious victim anything orally.
2. Do not induce vomiting unless told by medical personnel.
3. Do not give any medication to the victim unless directed by a doctor.
4. Do not neutralize the poison with lime juice/honey.

Prevention

For the prevention of poisoning some measures should be taken i.e. medicines, cleaning detergents, mosquito repellants and paints should be stored carefully. Keep all potentially poisonous substances out of children's reach. Label the poisons in your house. Avoid keeping poisonous plants in or around house. Take care while eating products such as berries, roots or mushrooms and teach children the need to exercise caution.

3. **Eye Poisoning:** Eye should be washed immediately with plenty of water for 5 minutes with eye lids open. Eye should not be rubbed and contact lenses, if worn, should be removed.

Treatment

A first-aid treatment kit for poisoning should be kept at home. The kit contains Syrup of Ipecac and Activated Charcoal. The kit must carry prominent instructions on the lid to call a doctor or the poison control unit of the nearby hospital.

(f) Heart diseases

Cardiac failure is a general term that refers to a condition in which heart is unable to perform the functions of delivery of nutrients to and removal of wastes from the cells. It may be acute or chronic. *Left ventricular failure* (LVF) may occur due to hypertension, coronary atherosclerosis or aortic valvar disease. *Right ventricular failure* (RVF) may occur due to certain diseases of the lungs, congestive heart failure or conditions which impede the blood flow into the right side of the heart.

Treatment

First-aid treatment in case of acute cardiac failure consists of preventing the onset of shock by the following methods:

1. By gentle handling of injured parts and by protecting from cold.
2. By prompt attention to the control of hemorrhage and pain.
3. By minimizing the loss of fluid from the body.
4. Early correction of dehydration and electrolyte loss.

Cardiac arrest signifies sudden cessation of effective circulation. First-aid treatment should be given within five minutes. The treatment consists of external cardiac massage together with mouth-to-mouth artificial respiration.

Heart attacks are caused by lack of blood supply to the heart. Sometimes attack may be sudden after physical exercise, emotional trauma etc. Patient feels pain in the left side of chest or back, which may radiate to left arm. He becomes ashen gray and absolutely pale, sweating and limbs may become cold and clammy.

A doctor should be called immediately. The patient should neither be disturbed nor allowed to stand up or walk around. Tight clothing, belt etc should be loosened. The patient should be transferred to a hospital or a doctor in a lying position.

RESUSCITATION METHODS

Resuscitation means revival from unconsciousness or apparent death, commonly known as **artificial respiration**. Resuscitation is an important first-aid treatment, which should be known to everybody. Commonly used resuscitation methods are described below:

(a) Back-Pressure-Arm-Lift Method

It is also known as the *Holger Nielson method* and is an effective technique for artificial respiration (Fig. 4.1). The injured person is placed facedown, elbows bent, arms overhead with one hand upon the other. The cheek is placed on the hand with face turned slightly to one side. Kneel on one knee at the head of the victim and put the foot of opposite leg near the elbow. Put your hands on the victim's back in such a way that the thumbs just touch, between the armpits. Rock slowly forward, elbow straight, until your arms are approximately vertical, exerting steady pressure upon the back of the chest. Rock back slowly sliding your hands to the victim's arms just above the elbows. Raise the arms until definite resistance is left from the victim's shoulders. Release the arms. This completes a full cycle and should be repeated at a rate of at least 12 times per minute.

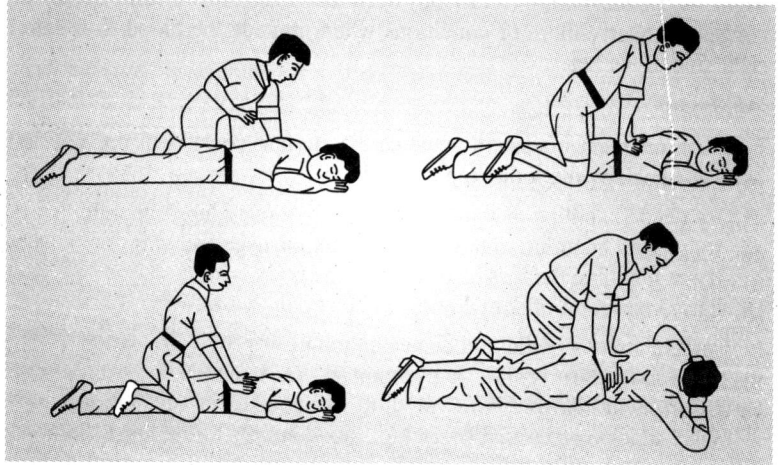

Fig. 4.1. Back-pressure-arm-lift method.

(b) Mouth to Mouth breathing Method

This method is most popular, simple and highly efficient. It is easily learnt and practiced. Small or young individuals can satisfactorily perform mouth-to-mouth breathing for an hour without undue fatigue, on subjects much larger than themselves. It can be done while the patient is being transported.

Steps: The victim should be laid on the back, his head held tilted back. The rescuer should take deep breath with mouth open widely and while keeping nostrils of the victim pinched; cover victim's mouth with his mouth smugly. Then watching the chest, blow into victim's lungs, until the chest blows up. Then withdraw the mouth, the chest should fall back. This should be repeated 15 to 20 times per minute. If the chest does not rise while blowing, then an obstruction should be looked for. If mouth-to-mouth respiration is not possible the mouth-to-nose respiration should be continued till normal breathing is restored (Fig. 4.2).

If the unconscious person is not breathing (asphyxia) then all clothing at waist, chest and neck should be loosened. The head of the victim should be tilted backward while supporting the back with rescuer's palm. This will clear the air passage of the victim and he may begin to breathe after a gasp. Even then if breathing does not start, movements of chest and lungs should be helped four or five times. This should be sufficient to start breathing. Failing this treatment also, mouth-to-mouth or mouth-to-nose respiration should be given.

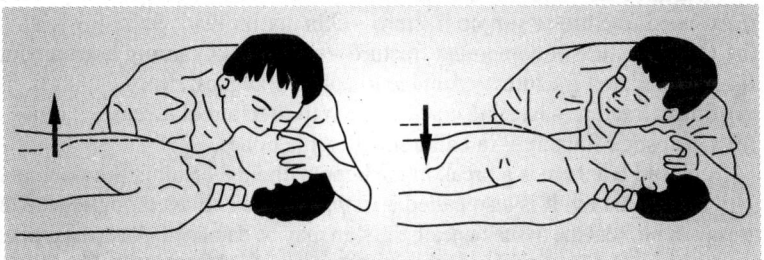

Fig. 4.2. Mouth-to-mouth breathing method

(c) External Heart Compression

This can be given when two trained persons are available. External heart compression goes along with artificial respiration. First-aider giving mouth-to-mouth respiration should sit to the right of the victim and second person should be on the left side. Second person should feel and mark the lower part of the sternum. He should place the heel of his hand (but not palm and fingers) on victim's chest and heel of the other hand over it. Then with his right arm the second person should press the sternum backwards towards the spine. Adults should be given about 60 pressures per minutes. Pupil will contract and carotid pulse will begin with each pressure (Fig. 4.3). If pulse is not restored then compression should be continued till the patient is transported to a hospital.

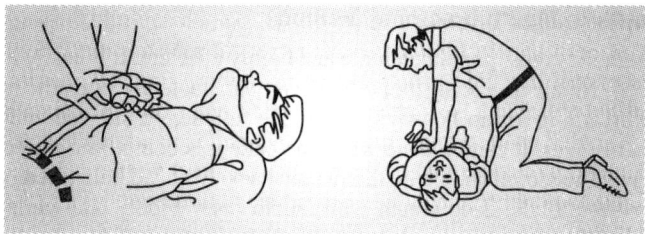

Fig. 4.3. External heart compression method.

FRACTURE

Fracture is a broken or cracked bone. It occurs when pressure is applied to bone. It occurs with/without displacement of bone fragments.

Accidents cause many different types of injuries to bones, joints and muscles. When rendering first-aid, one must be alert for signs of broken bones (fractures), dislocations, sprains, strains, and bruises (contusions). Injuries to the joints and muscles often occur together, and it is difficult to tell whether the injury is to a joint, muscle, or tendon. It is difficult to identify joint or muscle injuries from fractures. *When in doubt, always treat the injury as a fracture.*

Types

The fractures can be of following types:
(a) Closed fracture or simple fracture – skin not broken.
(b) Open fracture or compound fracture – skin breaks causing open wound.
(c) Complicated fractures – damage to adjacent organs.
(d) Stress fracture – hairline crack due to repeated stress.
(e) Greenstick fracture – in children's flexible bones.

A **closed fracture** is a break in the bone without a break in the skin i.e. the skin is not pierced. It is also called a *simple fracture*. Even though the skin is not cut or broken, the tissue beneath the skin may be damaged. An **open fracture** is a break in the bone with a break in the overlying skin as well. The break in the skin may be caused by the sharp end of the broken bone or by a foreign object such as a bullet or other thing penetrating the skin (Fig. 4.4). Thus when the bone is broken and there is a wound from the fracture to the skin surface then it is also called a **compound fracture**. *Open* or *compound fractures* are especially serious due to the danger of infection. Fracture may cause pain, loss of use of the limb or part, deformity, and swelling.

Signs and Symptoms of fracture

These include:
(a) severe pain,
(b) difficulty in movement,
(c) swelling/bruising/ bleeding,
(d) deformity/abnormal twist of limb, and
(e) tenderness on applying pressure.

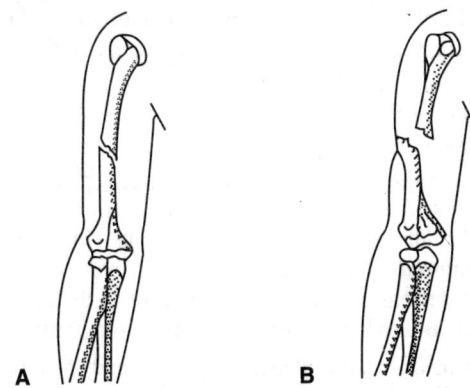

Fig. 4.4. Types of Fractures (A) Closed fracture, (B) Open fracture.

Treatment

It is not easy to recognize a fracture. All fractures, whether open or closed, can cause severe pain or shock. Fractures can cause the injured part to become deformed, or to take an unnatural position. Compare the injured to the uninjured part if you are unsure of a deformity. Pain, discoloration, and swelling may be at the fracture site, and there may be instability if the bone is broken clear through. It may be difficult or impossible for the casualty to move the injured part. If movement is possible, the casualty may feel a grating sensation (crepitus) as the ends of the bones rub against each other. If a bone is cracked rather than broken, the casualty may be able to move the injured part without much difficulty. An open fracture is easy to see if the end of the bone sticks out through the skin. If the bone does not stick out, one might see a wound but fail to see the broken bone. It can be difficult to tell if an injury is a fracture, dislocation, sprain, or strain. *When in doubt, apply splint.*

If a fracture is suspected, following **basic steps** should be followed:

1. Control bleeding with direct pressure, indirect pressure, or tourniquet only as a last resort.
2. Treat for shock.
3. Monitor the airway, breathing, and circulation (ABCs).
4. Remove all jewellery, if any, from the injury site, unless the casualty objects. Gently cut clothing away so that you don't move the injured part and cause further damage.
5. Check the distal pulse of the injured part; if pulse is absent, gently move injured part to restore circulation.
6. Cover all wounds with sterile dressings, including open fractures. Do not push bone ends back into the skin. Avoid excessive pressure on the wound.
7. Apply splint – *Do not attempt to straighten broken bones.*
   (a) Apply and maintain traction until the splint has been secured.
   (b) Wrap from the bottom of the splint to the top, firmly but not too tight.

(c) Check the distal pulse to ensure that circulation is still present. If the pulse is absent, loosen the splint until circulation returns. Do not move the casualty until the injury has been splinted.

8. Request for medical assistance – All suspected fractures require professional medical treatment.

The primary process of first-aid for fractures consists of immobilizing the injured part to prevent the ends of broken bones from moving and causing further damage to the nerves, blood vessels, or internal organs. Splints are also used to immunize injured joints or muscles and to prevent the enlargement of severe wounds. Before learning first-aid for injuries to the bones, joints, and muscles, one should need to have a general understanding of the use of splints.

First-aid treatment of fracture depends on type and location of fracture. First principle is '**splint them where they lie**'. Splints should be applied in simple fractures. A patient with a broken bone should never be moved until the break has been adequately splinted. If nothing else is available, rolled blankets or newspapers firmly bound in place can be used. In case of *compound fractures* the bleeding should be stopped first and the wound is bound by applying sterile gauge held in place by bandage or adhesive plaster and then splint is applied. Everything should be done carefully otherwise a *simple fracture* may be turned into a compound fracture.

Fixed traction type splints (Thomas Traction Splints) are recommended for fracture of the extremities but even padded blankets, umbrella or newspapers can also be used as splints. Wooden splints are easiest to handle. They should be long enough to reach beyond joints above and below fractures and always well padded. One splint on each side of the limb should be placed and bandaged. Absorbent cotton is the best for padding. The triangular or roller bandage or handkerchiefs, towels, garters, tapes, straps or adhesive plaster can be used for binding. Patient should be transported to a doctor's office only after he/she has been completely splinted, on a stretcher.

(a) Skull

In case of *skull fracture* the patient should be kept in reclining position with his head slightly raised and supported. Stimulants are not to be administered. If scalp wounds are present, sterile gauge should be applied and covered with a bandage. Patient must not be moved until adequate help is available.

The primary danger is that the brain may be damaged. Whether or not the skull is fractured is of secondary importance. The first-aid procedures are the same in both case, and the primary intent is to prevent further damage. Some injuries that fracture the skull do not cause brain damage but brain damage can result from minor injuries that do not cause damage to the skull.

It is difficult to determine whether an injury has affected the brain, because symptoms of brain damage vary. A victim who has suffered a head injury must be handled carefully and must be given immediate medical attention.

Signs and symptoms

Signs and symptoms that may indicate brain damage include wounds of the scalp, deformity of the skull, dizziness, weakness, conscious or unconscious, pain, tenderness or swelling, severe headache, nausea and vomiting, restlessness, confusion, disorientation, paralysis of the arms, legs, or face, unequal pupils, abnormal reaction to light. The other symptoms of skull fracture are blood or clear fluid from the ears, nose, or mouth; pale, flushed skin, bruising behind the ear (*Batlle's sign*) and bruising under or around the eyes in the absence of trauma to the eyes (*Raccoon's sign*).

Treatment

If you suspect a head injury, following steps should be taken:

(a) Position the casualty flat, stabilize the head and neck as you found them by placing your hands on both sides of the head.

(b) Establish and maintain an open airway-jaw-thrust maneuver. Note that the head is not tilted and the neck is not extended. Check the airway, breathing, and circulation (ABCs).

(c) Finger sweep to remove any foreign bodies from the mouth.

(d) Maintain neutral position of head and neck and, if possible, apply a cervical collar or improvised (towel) collar.

(e) Apply dressing – Do not use direct pressure or tie knots over the wound. Apply ice or cold packs if available (for blood or clear fluid from the nose or ears, cover loosely with a sterile dressing to absorb but not stop the flow).

(f) Treat for shock – Casualties with suspected head and neck injuries are to remain flat. *Do not raise the casualty's feet.* If they are vomiting or bleeding around the mouth, place them on their side keeping the neck straight. *Do not give anything to eat or drink.*

(g) Seek the medical assistance immediately – Head and neck injuries should be treated by professional medical personnel, if possible. *Do not attempt procedures that you are not trained to do.*

(b) Nasal bones

Injury should be covered with a gauze dressing held in place with a bandage or adhesive tape. Splint should not be attempted but patient taken to the physician.

(c) Lower jaw

Lower jaw should be brought to the upper and while holding in position apply either triangular or roller bandage around the chin to the top of the head (Fig. 4.5).

(d) Spine

The spinal column (also called as spine or backbone) consists of a series of bones called vertebrae. Always check for a spinal injury if the casualty has suffered a fall or has been hit in the back.

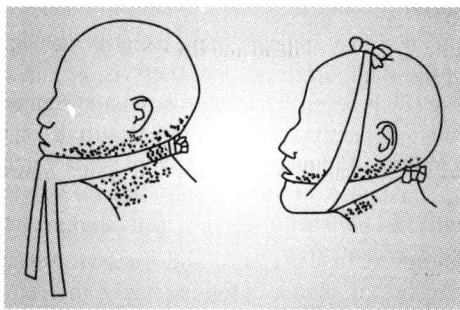

Fig. 4.5. Four-tailed bandage for a fractured jaw.

Signs and symptoms of an injured spine

These include:

1. Pain or tenderness of the neck or back.
2. Cut or bruise on the neck or back.
3. Inability to move part of the body (paralysis), especially the legs.
4. Lack of feeling in a body part.
5. Loss of bladder and/or bowel control.
6. Head or back in an unusual position.

Treatment

Patient should be moved to a hospital while preventing others from improperly moving him. If the patient has a broken neck, he must be transported on a rigid support, flat on his back, face up. If he is not already lying on his back, he must be turned into that position. If the patient has a broken back, he is transported in the face down position. If sufficient help or materials are not available to move the patient, cover him with a blanket and wait for adequate help. *It is better to do nothing than to do harm.* There should be available at least three persons to help so that the patient is put on the stretcher and transported without further harm (Fig. 4.6).

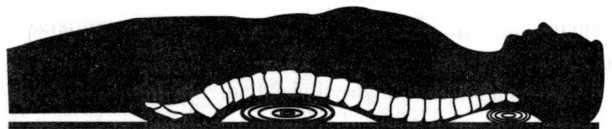

Fig. 4.6. Padding placed under back and neck.

In a nutshell, if a fractured spine is suspected, following **steps** should be taken:

(a) Position the casualty flat, stabilize the head and neck as you found them by placing your hands on both sides of the head.
(b) Establish and maintain an open airway-jaw-thrust maneuver. Note that the head is not tilted and the neck is not extended. Check the airway, breathing, and circulation (ABCs).

(c) Finger sweep to remove any foreign bodies from the mouth.

(d) Maintain neutral position of head and neck and, if possible, apply a cervical collar or improvised (towel) collar.

(e) Keep the casualty comfortable and warm enough to maintain normal body temperature.

(f) Treat for shock – Casualties with suspected spinal injuries are to remain flat. *Do not raise the casualty's feet.* If the casualty is vomiting or bleeding around the mouth, place them on their side keeping the neck straight. *Do not give anything to eat or drink.*

(g) Seek medical assistance immediately.

• *Do not move the casualty unless it is absolutely necessary.*

• *Do not bend or twist the casualty's body.*

• *Do not move the head forward, backward, or sideways. Do not allow the casualty to sit up.*

(e) Elbow

If the elbow is bent apply a sling to the elbow and bandage the arm to the body (Fig. 4.7 A and B). If the arm is straight, apply a well-padded splint on the front side and hold it in place with a bandage or adhesive plaster strips.

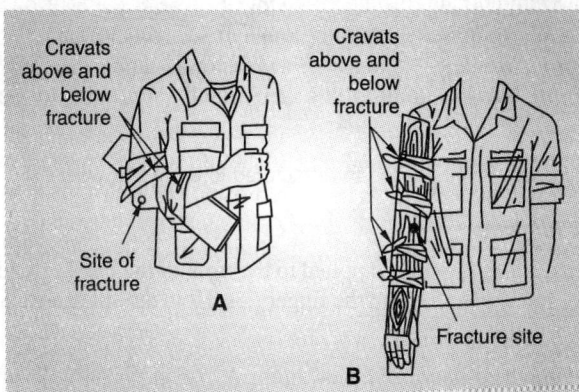

Fig. 4.7. Splint applied to a fractured elbow with (A) elbow bent, (B) arm straight.

(f) Upper arm

Bend the arm at the elbow and hold it close to the body. Tie a well-padded splint alongside the upper arm, reaching from the shoulder to the elbow or below. Place the forearm in a sling. Tie the arm to the side of the body with a wide bandage (Fig. 4.8).

(g) Forearm and Wrist

Two well-padded splints should be applied, one from the elbow to the finger tips on the front and another on the back of the forearm and hand. Splints are held in position with a bandage or adhesive plaster (Fig. 4.9).

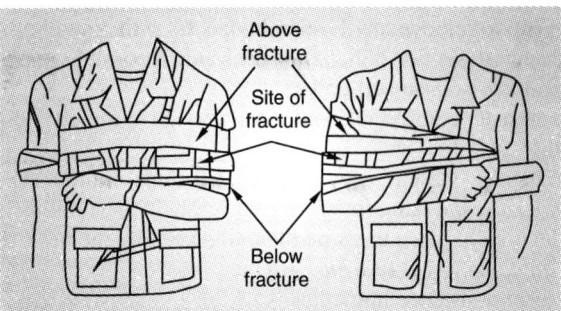

Fig. 4.8. Chest used as splint for an upper arm fracture.

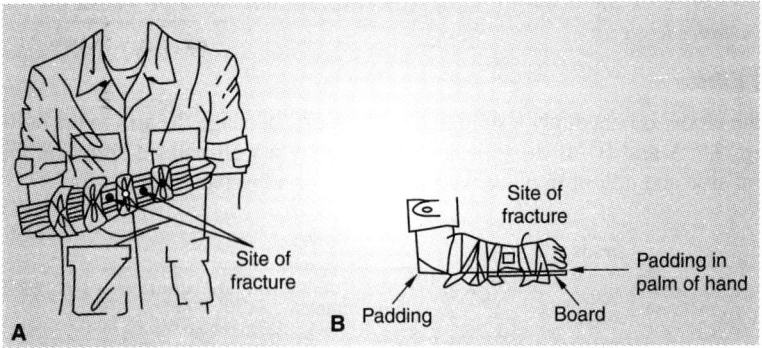

Fig. 4.9. Splint applied to a fractured forearm (A), wrist (B).

(i) Hand or Fingers

A well-padded splint should be applied to the front of the hand extending from the middle of forearm to beyond the finger tips. Hold the splint with a bandage and support it with a sling.

(j) Collar bone

The collar bone is also known as the clavicle. When standing, the injured shoulder is lower, and the casualty is unable to raise the arm above the shoulder. The casualty attempts to support the shoulder by holding the elbow. This is the typical stance taken by a casualty with a broken collar bone. Since the collar bone lies near the surface of the skin, you may be able to see the point of fracture by the deformity and tenderness.

In addition to the general procedures above, gently bend the victim's arm and place the forearm across the chest. The palm of the hand should be turned in, with the thumb pointing up. Support the arm in this position (Fig.4.10) with a wide sling. The hand should be raised about 4 inches above the level of the elbow. A wide roller bandage (or any wide strip of cloth) may be used to secure the victim's arm to the body.

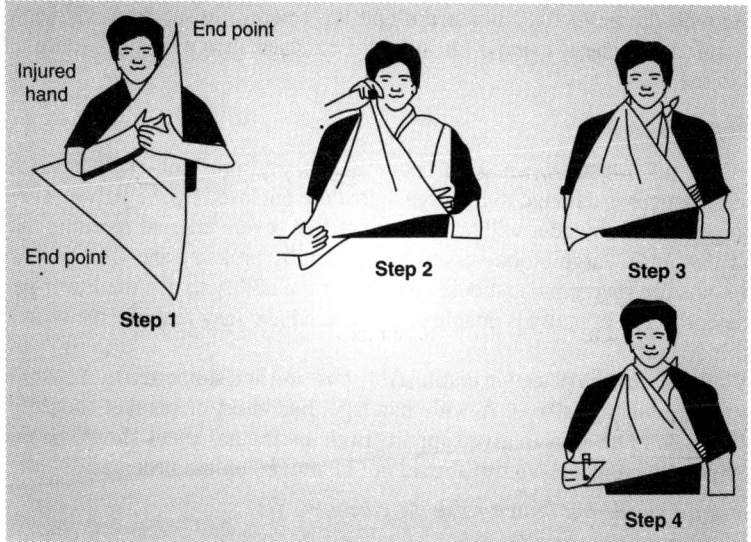

Fig. 4.10. Sling for immobilizing fractured collar bone.

(k) Ribs

Make the casualty as comfortable as possible so that the chances of further damage to the lungs, heart, or chest wall are minimized.

A common finding in all casualties with fractured ribs is pain at the site of the fracture. Ask the victim to point to the exact area of pain to assist you in determining the location of the fracture. Deep breathing, coughing, or movement is usually painful. The casualty should remain still and may lean toward the injured side with a hand over the fracture to immobilize the chest and ease the pain.

Simple rib fractures are not bound, strapped, or taped if the casualty is comfortable. If the casualty is more comfortable with the chest immobilized, use a sling and swathe (Fig. 4.11). Place the arm on the injured side against the

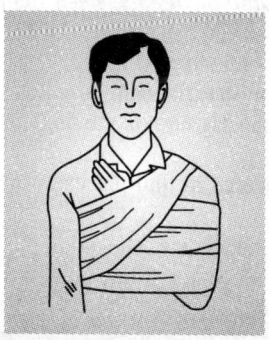

Fig. 4.11. Swathe bandage for fractured rib.

chest, with the palm flat, thumb up, and the forearm raised to a 45º angle. Immobilize the chest, using wide strips of bandage (ace wrap) to secure the arm to the chest.

(l) Pelvis (Hips)

Fractures often result from falls, heavy blows, and crushing accidents. The greatest danger is damage to the organs that are enclosed by the pelvis. There is danger that the bladder will be ruptured or that severe internal bleeding may occur due to the large blood vessels being torn by broken bone. The primary symptoms are severe pain, shock, and loss of the ability to use the lower part of the body. The casualty is unable to sit or stand and may feel like the body is "coming apart."

Victim should be placed in comfortable position and supported by a cushion under and around his hips. A wide bandage, bed sheet or blanket should be applied around his hips to give support. Both ankles and knees should be tied together with bandage. Victim should not be moved unless necessary.

- *Treat for shock, but do not raise the casualty's feet.*
- *Do not move the casualty unless absolutely necessary.*
- *Seek medical assistance asap (as early as possible).*

(m) Thigh

Grasp the injured limb at the heel and pull gently so that it is brought in line with the body. Apply two well-padded splints, a longer one outside extending from the armpit to the foot, the inner one from the crotch to the foot. Fasten splints with bandage around waist, hips, crotch, above and below knee, and at the ankle. If only one splint is available, it should be applied to the outside. Place cushion or pillow between the thigh and legs, and tie the two limbs together. The splint should be secured in five places: (a) around the ankle, (b) over the knee, (c) just below the hip, (d) around the pelvis, and (e) just below the armpit (Fig. 4.12). The legs can then be tied together to support the injured leg.

- *Do not move the victim until the leg has been splinted.*

(n) Knee-cap

The injured limb should be straightened. A splint should be applied on the back of the leg reaching from high up on the thigh to the heel (Fig 4.13 A and B).

The splint should be secured in four places:

1. Just below the hip.
2. Just above the knee.
3. Just below the knee.
4. Just above the ankle.

- *Do not place the straps directly over the kneecap.*

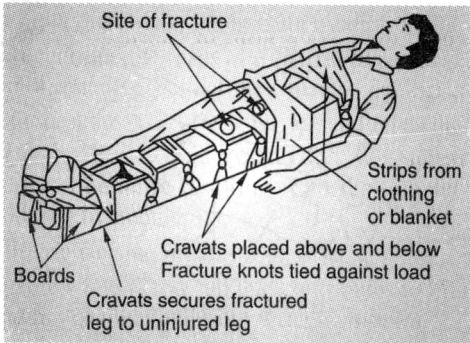

Fig. 4.12. Splint applied to a fractured thigh.

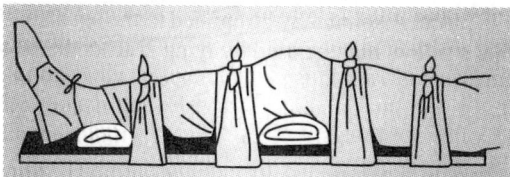

Fig. 4.13 A. Immobilization of fractured kneecap.

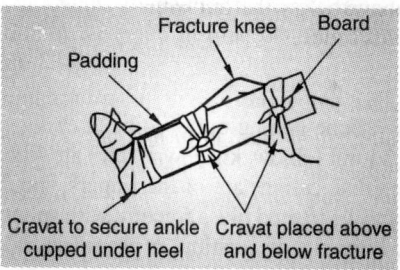

Fig. 4.13 B. Splint applied to a fractured knee.

(o) Leg

Gently grasp the leg and pull it in line with the body, apply two board splints to the side of the injured leg reaching from above the knee down to a point below the heel (Fig. 4.14). If only one splint is available it should be applied to outside of the leg and both legs bound together. If wooden splint is not available, a pillow may be placed under the limb and tied around the leg. A combination pillow and outside board splint can also be used. If none of these is available then the injured limb may be tied with bandages to healthy limb.

(p) Bones of the foot

Remove the shoes and stockings, if necessary by cutting them. Apply a well-padded splint to sole of the foot, extending from the heel to a little beyond the

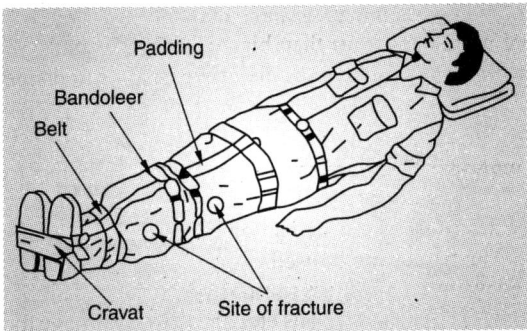

Fig. 4.14. Splint applied to a fractured leg.

toes and tie it in place. A splint may be applied to the leg also. If wooden splint is not available, a pillow may be used by tying it around the foot and ankle.

Precautions

Do not do the following things:

1. Massage the affected area.
2. Straighten the broken bone.
3. Move without support to broken bone.
4. Move joints above/below the fracture.
5. Give oral liquids/food.

(q) Dislocation

Dislocation means a bone getting out of joint. A *dislocation* occurs when the bones comprising a joint (elbow, knee, wrist etc) are forced out of their proper positions. Common dislocations are of the fingers, shoulders, jaw, elbow and hip. A dislocation can be treated like a fracture with splints or sling. No attempt should be made to correct a dislocation. A physician should be called.

(r) Sprain

A sprain results when a joint is twisted beyond its normal limits of motion and the connecting tissues around the joint tear. A sprain can produce signs and symptoms similar to those of a fracture and should be treated as a fracture of the joint.

ELEMENTS OF SURGERY

Surgery is the science and practice of treating injuries and diseases by operations. Management of wounds is the most important aspect of surgery. From the earliest times the healing of wounds has been the central problem in surgical practice.

A **wound** is caused when any tissue of the body e.g. skin, muscle, bone etc is torn or cut by injury. Bleeding normally occurs from a wound. The depth of a wound is more important than its area. Small deep wounds caused by knives, bullets etc are more dangerous than bigger surface wounds. A wound on the surface of the body or skin exposes the deeper tissues to danger of sepsis.

(a) Types of wounds

1. **Incised wounds:** These are caused by sharp instruments like knife, razor, glass etc. These wounds bleed very much.
2. **Contused wounds:** These are caused by blows by blunt instruments or by crushing. The tissues are bruised.
3. **Lacerated wounds:** These are caused by machinery, falls of rough surfaces, pieces of shells, claw of animals etc. These wounds have torn and irregular edges but they bleed less. Such wounds are most common in road traffic accidents. They are frequently dirty and contaminated with organic matter.
4. **Punctured wounds:** These are caused by stabs by any sharp instrument like a knife or a dagger. They have small openings but may be very deep hence more dangerous.

(b) First-aid treatment of wounds

Wounds cause two dangers, (i) bleeding, and (ii) infection. Hence the aim of first-aid is to stop bleeding and prevent infection. Bleeding is the immediate danger and should be treated promptly. To stop bleeding, direct pressure should be applied to the wound with a sterile dressing or a clean handkerchief. Arterial pressure should be pressed, if necessary. Any foreign object like glass, stones etc should be removed, if possible without opening the wound, else more bleeding may be caused. The wound should be covered with a clean dressing and bandaged firmly. A doctor or nurse should be approached and the wound should be treated within 6 to 8 hours. Complete healing of wounds takes a long time, sometimes a year or two.

DRESSINGS

A **dressing** is a protective covering applied to a wound. The **functions** of a dressing are (i) to prevent infection, (ii) to absorb discharge, (iii) to control bleeding, and (iv) to avoid further injury. An efficient dressing should be sterile and have a high degree of porosity to allow for oozing and sweating.

A. Classification of Dressings

(a) Primary wound dressing

These dressings are placed next to a wound surface. The function of primary wound dressing is to absorb the wound secretion and minimize maceration. The dressing consists of layers of gauze or any other clean, soft, absorbent material like linen. Absorbent cotton, bandages and similar materials should never be used directly on a wound surface as primary dressing.

A quick drying aerosol spray that forms a clear, plastic film is available as *Healex Spray* (Rallis India Ltd). The spray forms a smooth, transparent protective film which is insoluble in water or body fluids. It is easily removed without pain and is useful in minor surgery, small abrasions etc.

OASIS Ultra Tri-Layer Matrix is a natural extracellular matrix (ECM) derived from three layers of porcine small intestinal submucosa (SIS) technology. The three-layer construct of OASIS Ultra is designed to provide increased thickness, strength, and durability. Increased strength and thickness allow for easier fixation, including sutures and staples. Its features are- i) layers of bioresorbable extracellular matrix bring increased structure into the wound, ii) uses SIS technology to help replace and repair damaged tissues, iii) extra thickness offers easier handling and application, iv) retains key collagen and non-collagen components, v) comes ready to apply to save on preparation time, (vi) easy to trim to exact size and shape of wound, and (vi) minimally processed and sterilized.

Convatec Aquacel Hydrofiber dressing is a sterile, white, fibrous dressing derived from 100% pure sodium carboxymethylcellulose (NaCMC). *Aquacel* combines the look, feel, and handling properties of gauze and leading alginates, but retains more fluid than alginates and almost three times more fluid than gauze when used under compression. *Aquacel Hydrofiber Dressing* is indicated for the management of pressure ulcers, leg ulcers, abrasions, lacerations, incisions, donor sites and second degree burns and on infected wounds; for use in managing surgical or traumatic wounds that have been left to heal by secondary intention. Additionally, it can be used on wounds prone to bleeding and to facilitate the control of minor bleeding. The main features of *Aquacel Hydrofiber Dressing* are: (i) favorable gelling characteristics, (ii) contains antimicrobial ionic silver, and (iii) for moderate to high exudate wounds.

(b) Absorbents

Surgical cotton is the basic absorbent. Absorbent cotton is prepared from the raw cotton fiber and is free from natural waxes, impurities and foreign substances.

Surgical gauze is also prepared from raw cotton. It provides an absorbent material of sufficient tensile strength for surgical dressings.

(c) Bandages

These are made from flannel, calico, elastic net or special paper. The function of bandages is to hold dressings in place or to provide slight pressure or support. They may be elastic or inelastic. Triangular bandages and roller bandages are most commonly used.

(d) Adhesive tape

Main use of adhesive tape is to pull something into place and then hold it there. It is also used to affix something in place, as a protective covering for dressings. Small blisters, certain skin lesions and many wounds can be covered and protected from contamination by the proper use of tape. A variety of adhesive tapes are available in the market.

(e) Protective

These are used to cover wet dressings and hot or cold compresses. They are also used as a covering for poultices, and for the retention of heat. They prevent the escape of moisture from the dressings or compresses. Protective in common use are plastic sheeting, rubber sheeting and waxed or paraffined paper.

Surgical dressings must be stored and used with great care so as to maintain their sterility otherwise they may transmit infection.

Environment and Health

INTRODUCTION

State of positive health means a state of complete physical, mental and moral well being of individuals. This requires a balance of the internal environment of a man himself and the external environment in which he lives. Very frequently the key to the nature, occurrence, prevention and control of diseases lies in the environment.

Environment means the air, water, and land in which people, animals, and plants live.

Sanitation is the science of *safeguarding* health. Environmental sanitation is defined as 'the control of all those factors in man's physical environment, which may cause a deleterious effect on his physical development, health and survival'. The term sanitation covers the whole field of controlling the environment with an aim to prevent diseases and promote health. Besides food, water, housing and clothing, sanitation is an important factor in the environment. Improper sanitation, non-availability of adequate safe water and its disposal, air pollution, industrial pollution and increasing population all are posing serious threats to the healthy environment. Therefore attainment of a healthy environment is becoming more and more complex.

India is still lagging behind many countries in the field of environmental health. The basic problem of safe water supply and sanitary disposal of human excreta still pose a serious challenge before the country.

WATER

There is no life without water. This is the reason why man preferred to settle near water sources i.e. near rivers, lakes etc. Water is the essential and predominant constituent of living cell protoplasm. It is a necessary vehicle for all the metabolic processes. Water constitutes nearly two thirds of the total body weight, 79% of blood, 80% of brain and 10% of bones. It is required for domestic, public, agricultural and individual purposes. Supply of safe and potable drinking water to the country is of greatest importance in maintaining positive health measures. *Safe water* is one that cannot harm the consumer. Drinking water should not only be safe but also agreeable to use. Such water is called *potable water*. Thus the desirable qualities of safe, potable water should include freedom from pathogenic agents, freedom from harmful substances, pleasant to taste and usable for domestic purposes. On an average every individual should be supplied with 150 to 200 liters of water every day.

A. Sources of Water Supply

All water is primarily derived from ocean. In topical regions about 700 gallons of water are evaporated every minute from every square mile of ocean surface. Evaporated water reaches the earth back in the form of rain, hail, snow, dew or mist. This condensed water from the air is the ultimate source of all our natural water supply. On reaching earth a part of rainwater is evaporated again into the atmosphere, some part gets collected in the form of lakes, ponds, etc. A major part of it runs away in the direction of natural slope of ground and gets collected in the form of small streams which form rivers and finally runs into the sea and thus the hydrological cycle goes on. This is explained in Fig.5.1.

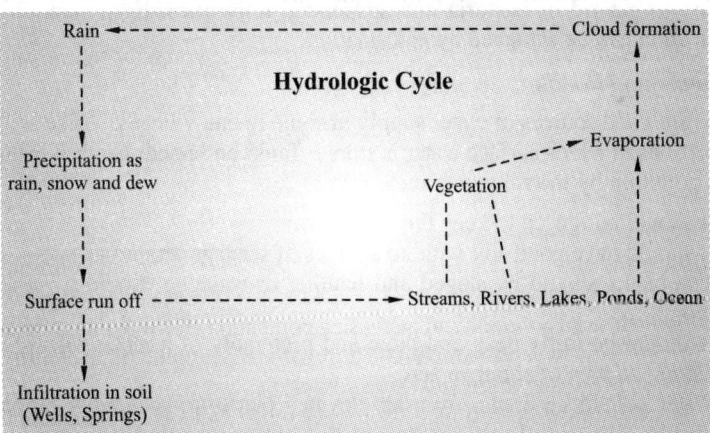

Fig. 5.1. Hydrological cycle and sources of water.

Main Sources of Water Supply

(a) Rain Water

Rain water is not an important source of water supply in the world except in Malta and Gibraltar. It is the purest form of water but receives impurities from the atmosphere during its fall to earth e.g. dust, soot, suspended matter, microbes, gases like hydrogen sulfide, carbon dioxide, ammonia, nitrogen, oxygen etc.

Properly collected and stored rain water is safe. It is useful for cooking, washing and bathing purposes. However rain water being soft, it is liable to corrode lead pipes and may cause lead poisoning. This drawback can be overcome by using an alternate to lead pipes. A rainfall of 1" corresponds to about 21.25 liters on one square yard of land.

(b) Surface Water

It is the water which drains from the surface, for example, rain water reaching the ground or flowing of melted snow from hills, seen as a river, canal, stream, lake or a pond. In India many cities like Delhi, Kolkata and Ahmedabad depend on river water for their needs. River water is fairly pure and unpolluted at its source but becomes polluted during its course as most rivers and streams serve as the natural sewer of the region they drain. The river water is grossly contaminated and it is quite unfit for drinking without treatment. Since flowing water possesses 'self purification' action, the running water in rivers, canals and streams is generally purified to a certain extent. The impurities are removed due to oxidation by oxygen dissolved in water, absorption of organic impurities by vegetable and animal life e.g. fish etc, settling of solid matter due to gravitation and dilution by the tributaries etc. The sun too has a purifying action. Water collected from the river at least 20 to 30 feet away from the bank is least contaminated.

To protect against contamination, water from a river, canal or stream should be collected in large reservoirs or settling tanks. Such stored water can be filtered to get rid of bacteria and suspended impurities. High standard of purification can be achieved by chlorination.

(c) Tanks and Ponds

These are good sources of water supply in some Indian villages. These are the excavations in which surface water is stored. Tanks and ponds can be kept free from pollution by the following measures:

1. It should be fenced to keep the cattle away.
2. It should have good soil with no sources of seepage around its site.
3. The banks should be sloped and bathing or washing should be strictly prohibited.
4. It should be fairly deep and large and preferably of a rectangular shape having an area of about an acre.
5. Water should be drawn from an elevated platform, preferably by hand pumps.
6. Any trade like jute steeping should not be allowed in the tanks.
7. Weeds and algae should be periodically removed and Gambusia fish kept to eat away the larvae.

Lakes are natural collection of surface water or upland surface water.

(d) Upland Water

It is the water which runs on the sides of hills, slopes and valleys and is collected in artificially made lakes (catchment areas). Water may be collected in the form of natural lakes as in the city of Glasgow or in artificially constructed lakes as in cities like Mumbai, Chennai and Darjeeling. In Shimla it is collected at *Mahasu* ridge. In Mumbai there are four lakes for this purpose i.e. *Vihar* lake, *Tulsi* lake, *Tansa* lake and *Vaitarna* lake. Upland surface water is safe because it is pure rainwater.

The **sources of impurities** in water are: (i) contamination from human and animal excreta, which can be prevented by strict prohibition, (ii) lead poisoning due to softness of rain water, which can be avoided by using other pipes, (iii) in some areas the ground water contains peat, a decayed vegetable matter, which makes water acidic and causes diarrhoea symptoms. This can be avoided by discouraging vegetation around such areas.

Because of the chances of contamination due to the reasons mentioned above, upland surface water should be purified by filtration and treated with chlorine or simply by running through a bed of fine sand, before final storage.

E. Pole's formula can be used to calculate the yield of the catchment area.

$$Q = 62.15A\ (4/5\ R - E)$$

where Q is the volume of water in gallons, A is the area in acres, R is the average rainfall for three driest consecutive years, and E is loss in inches by evaporation.

(e) Ground Water

It is the cheapest and most practical means of providing water to communities. It is superior to surface water because the ground acts as an effective filter medium for water. Water gets filtered and purified while passing over it. The advantages of ground water are:

1. It is usually free from pathogenic agents.
2. It usually requires no further treatment.
3. The supply is nearly assured even during dry seasons.

The disadvantages include high mineral content, which render the water hard, and need for pumping to lift the water.

Sources of ground water are springs and wells.

(a) **Wells:** Wells are artificially driven holes to reach the underground water level. They are the main source of water supply in Indian villages. Wells are of four varieties:

(i) **Shallow wells:** These simply tap the subsoil water i.e. ground water lying between the surface and first impermeable strata. The term 'shallow' has nothing to do with the depth of the well. The water of these wells gets easily polluted from surface with sewage and other impurities from surrounding cesspools, leaking drains, privies, droppings of animal and plant leaves. It is an unsafe source of water and chemically water is moderately hard. Most of the wells in India are of this type.

(ii) **Deep wells:** Deep well is dug well, which goes beyond the first impervious layer to reach the water strata below. The water is comparatively safer for drinking purposes than shallow wells. This is due to efficient filtration because the water travels a greater distance through the earth and also gets better protection from surface contamination. The water is much harder due to nitrites and nitrates.

(iii) **Artesian wells:** These are a variety of deep wells in which water under great pressure comes out to the surface automatically. The strata are cup-shaped and surface of well is much lower than the upper layer of water stratum tapped. They derive their name after *Artois* province in France where they have been in use for a very long time. These wells are not common in India.

(iv) **Tube wells:** These are shallow wells formed by simply driving galvanized iron pipes (1.5 to 2″ diameter and 20 to 25′ deep) to trap the ground water. A pump is attached to the pipe to draw the water. These are more sanitary than the dug wells. The water is bacteriologically safe and cheaper in comparison to other sources. These wells are successful as a source of drinking water in many parts of India. The entire water supply in Chandigarh is through tube wells. Different varieties of wells are shown in Fig. 5.2.

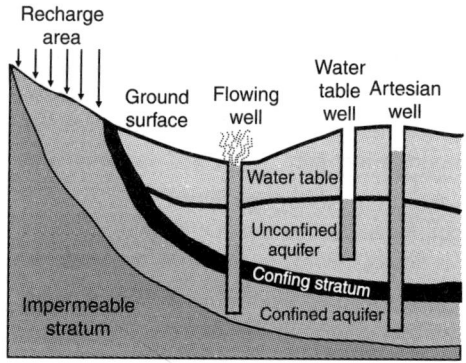

Fig. 5.2. Varieties of wells.

(b) **Springs:** These are natural outlets of ground water held under pressure by the impermeable layer. The quality and quantity of water from springs is unreliable. Springs are not considered as an important source of water supply because their yield is very low. In India springs are an unimportant source of water supply. Springs are of following types:

(i) **Shallow or Surface or Land Springs:** They issue from superficial water-bearing sand or gravel and reach the surface at the foot of the slopes. They resemble shallow wells.

(ii) **Deep or Main Springs:** They issue at points of outcrops from porous strata located between impervious strata. They resemble deep wells.

(iii) **Hot or Thermal Springs:** They issue from regions where volcanic eruptions have ceased and they have high temperature.

(iv) **Mineral Springs:** The water of these springs contains minerals like sulfur, iron, magnesium etc hence these are called mineral springs. Spring water is usually hard and unfit for washing.

WATER POLLUTION

Water pollution is a serious problem in India. The common impurities polluting water are described below.

A. Inorganic Impurities

Suspended impurities

These include sand, mud, silt, chalk etc and can be removed by sedimentation or alum precipitation. These impurities cause mechanical irritation of gastrointestinal tract and even diarrhoea.

Dissolved impurities

1. Gases e.g. CO_2 and H_2S, which make water acidic.
2. Salts e.g. carbonates, chlorides, calcium and magnesium sulfate. These produce temporary and permanent hardness. Hard water may cause dyspepsia and diarrhoea and also difficulty in cooking and washing.
3. Iron resulting from rusting of pipes. It produces dyspepsia and constipation
4. Zinc, which causes constipation.
5. Lead, which causes lead poisoning.
6. Fluorine, which causes fluorosis and enamel mottling.

B. Organic Impurities

Organic impurities are due to:

1. Human activities: sewage, which contains decomposable organic matter and pathogenic agents.
2. Refuse, house waste and droppings.
3. Industrial and trade wastes, which contain toxic agents like synthetic organic chemicals.

   Use of polluted water is hazardous.

Hazards of Polluted Water

These are of two types:

1. Biological Hazards

These comprise of water-borne diseases. About 500 million people are affected by these diseases every year in the world, In India about 2 million deaths occur due to water-borne diseases every year.

Water-borne diseases	
Agent	*Diseases caused*
Viral	Infective hepatitis, Poliomyelitis, Gastroenteritis
Bacterial	Diarrhoea, Dysentery, Cholera, Enteric fever, Gastroenteritis, Typhoid and Paratyphoid
Protozoal	Amoebiasis, Giardiasis
Helminthic	Round worm, Whipworm, Threadworm, Hydated diseases
Spirochetal	Weil's disease
Through Cyclops	Guinea worm infection
Through snails	Schistosomiasis

2. Chemical Hazards

Chemical pollutants include acids, dyes, detergents, solvents, cyanides, heavy metals, nitrogenous substances, leaching agents, pigments and other toxic substances. Some contaminants like pesticides, herbicides, fungicides, polymers, plastic ingredients and heavy metals are carcinogenic and mutagenic.

The "Prevention and Control of Water Pollution Act, 1974" was passed by the Parliament to safeguard against these serious hazards of polluted water. Several other legislations have also been implemented in this regard.

WATER PURIFICATION

Large-scale purification of water is necessary for public use because it makes the water free from most of the common impurities. Water of highest purity is used in the manufacture of parenteral preparations in the pharmaceutical industry.

The steps involved in the large scale purification of water are:

1. Aeration and purification
2. Chlorination
3. Filtration
4. Storage and distribution

In *aeration* process, oxygen mixes with water and gases like CO_2 and H_2S are expelled. If water is stored in a reservoir for about a month, it may purify itself. Over 90% impurities settle by gravitation in four hours. The factors concerned in the purification of water are temperature, sunlight, velocity of water flow and the purpose for which actions take place.

Coagulation is necessary, especially for muddy water of river, prior to rapid sand filtration.

Filtration removes suspended impurities, bacteria, ova and cysts from the water. Two types of filters are commonly used; *(i)* the 'biological' or 'slow sand' filters, and *(ii)* the 'mechanical' or 'rapid sand' filters. A detailed comparison between slow sand filters and rapid sand filters is described in Table 5.1.

A. Slow Sand Filtration

Slow sand filters were first introduced in England in 1804 and hence this system of filtration is also called 'English system'. Initial cost of construction of water-proof filter bed is higher than rapid sand filters but maintenance cost is low. Essential elements of a slow sand filter are described below (Fig. 5.3).

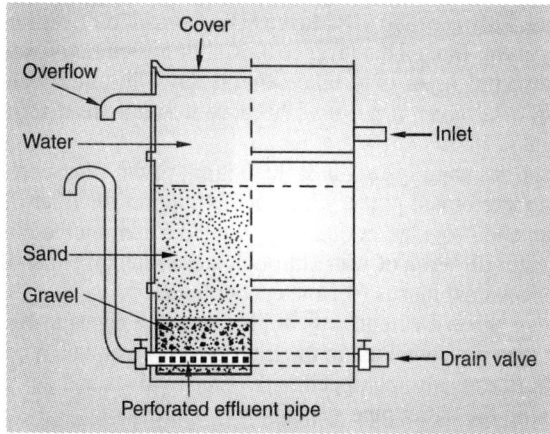

Fig. 5.3. Schematic diagram of a Slow Sand Filter.

(a) Supernatant raw water
(b) Graded sand bed
(c) Underdrainage system
(d) System of filter control valves

The raw water from the source is collected and stored in large open reservoirs (settling tanks) for 24 to 48 hours. This allows sedimentation of suspended matter. The process of sedimentation can be accelerated by use of coagulants such as alum. This treatment reduces the bacterial count of water by 90%. It also serves the purpose of maintaining a constant head of water over the sand bed and facilitates downward flow of water through the sand filter. The processes of sedimentation, oxidation and agglomeration of particles also take place. Supernatant water is always maintained at a constant level.

The total depth of the filter is about 3.6 meters and various levels from top to bottom are as follows:

Water on top	1.5 to 1.8 meters
Under drain	2 layered bricks
Gravel	15 to 30 cm
Coarse sand	15 to 30 cm
Fine sand	0.6 to 0.9 meters

Sand bed is the most vital part of the filter and presents a large surface area. One cubic meter of sand has an area of 15000 sq. meters. While water percolates slowly through the sand bed, it is subjected to various purification processes such as mechanical straining, sedimentation, adsorption, oxidation and bacterial action.

Real biological action occurs in the vital layer. After the filter bed has been working for 2 to 3 days; a thin, green slimy gelatinous layer of low vegetable organic thread-like algae and fungi etc is formed on the surface of the superficial layer of sand. This is called **vital layer**. The formation of vital layer is known as *ripening* of the filter. This layer retains all the bacteria of water. Complete formation of vital layer may take several days. Filtered water before the formation of vital layer is not used because it is not freed from most of the biological impurities.

The under-drainage system is at the bottom of the filter bed. It consists of the porous or perforated pipes, which act as support for filter medium above on one hand, and provides an outlet for filtered water, on the other hand.

For efficient filtration of water through these filters the rate of flow should not exceed 4 vertical inches (0.1 meter) per hour.

The above three elements e.g. supernatant water, sand bed and under-drainage system are contained in the filter box. To maintain a constant rate of filtration the filter is also equipped with certain valves and devices which are incorporated in the outlet pipe system.

Slow sand filters can reduce the total bacterial counts of water by 99.99%.

B. Rapid Sand Filtration

This system is most commonly used for muddy river waters whose average turbidity is between 10 to 30 ppm. Water filtration rate through these filters is very high – 5 to 15 cubic meter/sq. metre/hour; about 40 to 50 times more than that of slow sand filters. The initial cost of construction and space requirement is much more than slow sand filters but the maintenance cost is relatively higher.

The steps involved in the process of rapid filtration are shown in Fig. 5.4.

Rapid sand filters may be of two types:

1. Pressure type e.g. Candy's filter
2. Gravity type e.g. Paterson's filter is the most important rapid filter.

Paterson's Rapid Filter

The raw water is pumped into settling tanks and is led continuously into the plant after passing through the measuring gear. A coagulant, usually alum (5 to

Table 5.1 Comparison between Slow sand filter and Rapid sand filter

Item	Slow Sand Filter	Rapid Sand Filter
Pre-treatment	Not required except plain sedimentation	Coagulation, flocculation and sedimentation
Base materials	Gravel base of 30 to 75 cm depth with 3 to 65 mm size graded gravel	Gravel base of 45 to 50 cm depth with gravel size varies from 3 to 50 mm in 4 or 5 layers
Filter sand		
• Effective size	• 0.25 to 0.35 mm	• 0.45 to 0.70 mm
• Uniformity coefficient	• 3.0 to 5.0	• 1.2 to 1.7
• Thickness of sand bed	• 80 to 100 cm	• 60 to 75 cm
Under drainage system	Open-jointed pipes or drains covered with perforated blocks	Perforated pipe laterals discharging into main header
Size of each unit	50 to 200 sq. m	10 to 100 sq. m
Rate of filtration	100 to 200 Lit/hr/sq. m	4800 to 7200 Lit/hr/sq. m
Cost		
• Installation	• High	• Low
• O & M	• Low	• High
Efficiency		
• Turbidity of feed water	Low; < 30 Net Turbidity Units (NTU)	Any level of turbidity of feed water (with pre-treatment)
• Removal of bacteria	98 to 99%	80 to 90%
Suitability	For water supply to rural areas and small towns	For public water supply to towns and cities
Post-treatment	Slight disinfection	Complete disinfection is a must
Ease of construction	Simple	Complicated
Skilled supervision	Not essential	Essential
Loss of head		
• Initial	• 10 cm	• 30 cm
• Final	• 80 to 120 cm	• 250 to 350 cm
Method of cleaning	• Scrapping and removing 1.5 to 3 cm thick sand layer • Laborious	• Back washing with or without compressed air agitation • Simple and easy
Quantity of wash water required	0.2 to 0.5% of total water filtered	1 to 5% of total water filtered
Cleaning interval	Three to four months	One to two days

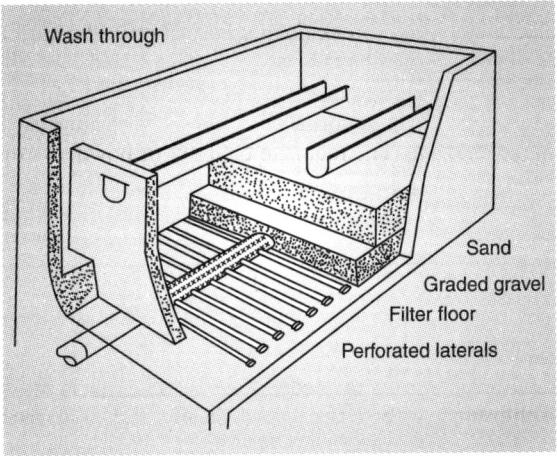

Fig. 5.4. Schematic diagram of a Rapid sand filter.

40 mg/liter of water, is added). While flowing through the trough the water is mixed with the chemical by means of baffle plate and reacts with calcium carbonate, and a flocculent white gelatinous precipitate of aluminum hydroxide is formed.

$$Al_2(SO_4) + 3\ Ca\ (HCO_3)_2 = Al_2(OH)_6 + 3CaSO_4 + 6CO_2$$

Water enters into another tank where suspended and colloidal matters get precipitated. Flocculent precipitate also settles down and carries other suspended matter and bacteria present in water. This also reduces load on filters. After this stage water is admitted to a series of rapid filters.

The alum-flock not removed by sedimentation is held back on the sand bed and forms a slimy layer on the surface of the sand though which water is forced. Adsorption of bacteria and oxidation of ammonia also take place during filtration.

From the filters, water is passed into a chlorinating chamber where chlorine gas is added. Chlorine exerts its germicidal action; oxidizes iron, magnesium and hydrogen sulfide; controls algae formation; and helps in coagulation.

Gradually filters get clogged with bacteria and impurities, and their efficiency falls. When loss of water approaches 7 to 8 feet, the filters are subjected to a washing action (back washing).

C. Chlorination

It is most efficient, cheap, reliable and easily available method of water purification. Chlorine may be used in the form of gas or solution or as bleaching powder. Chlorine kills pathogenic bacteria (but doesn't affect spores and viruses), oxidizes iron, manganese and hydrogen sulfide, destroys some taste and odour-producing constituents, controls algae and slime organisms, and helps in coagulation.

The point at which free chlorine (i.e. chlorine demand of water) begins to appear is called *break point* (break point chlorination). The chlorine left after this point is called *residual chlorine,* which acts as a disinfectant.

Bleaching powder or chlorinated lime is white amorphous powder or brittle lumps having a faint odour of chlorine and disagreeable saline taste. It contains 33% of available chlorine. The requisite quantity of powder is dissolved and mixed with water in a mixing tank. The mixture is allowed to flow into a storage tank and taken to the main water supply. In India bleaching powder is largely used for sterilizing wells, tanks, canals or rivers, especially when cholera spreads in the rural areas.

Dosage of chlorine

Filtered water supply can be sterilized by 0.25 parts of chlorine per million parts of water. More quantity is needed if organic matter is present in water. For effective chlorination, the free residual chlorine should be 0.1 to 0.2 ppm. The dosage is controlled with chlorinator. The minimum recommended concentration of free chlorine is 0.5 mg per liter for one hour.

Superchlorination and Dechlorination

Superchlorination requires 2 parts of free chlorine per million gallons of water for 15 minutes instead of 1ppm of chlorine for 30 minutes. Excess of chlorine is neutralized (dechlorination) by adding 9.5 g of sodium thiosulphate per 450 liters of water. This process removes possible unpleasant taste of water. The method is applicable to heavily polluted waters of greatly varying quality.

Horrock's Test

This test is employed to calculate the quantity of bleaching powder needed for effective sterilization of given volume of water.

The Horrock's apparatus consists of a black cup (for standard bleaching powder), 6 white cups for water to be tested and cadmium iodide plus starch solution as indicator. All white cups are filled with water and one drop of standard bleaching powder solution (prepared in black cup) is added to cup No. 1, 2 drops in cup No. 2, 6 drops in cup No. 6. This is mixed and allowed to stand for 30 minutes and then a drop of indicator is added to each cup. The number of cup showing blue colour indicates the number of scoops (equal to 2g) of bleaching powder to give one part of free chlorine per 100 gallons of water at the end of half an hour contact period with that water.

Iodine Test

This test is used for determination of residual chlorine. 1 to 2 drops of starch solution is added in chlorinated water followed by a drop of iodine solution. A blue colour develops if free chlorine is present in water.

Orthotoludine Test

This is a test for assessing the effectiveness of chlorination. To 10 mL of chlorinated water, 10 drops of orthotoludine solution is added in a test tube.

Development of immediate yellow colour (flash test) indicates just sufficient chlorination, red colour after some time means excess of chlorination due to chloramine.

D. Domestic Purification of Water

For small scale and domestic purification of water the following methods are useful: boiling, distillation, filtration through muslin cloth, charcoal, sand etc, three pitchers method and domestic filters. Only domestic filters are described below because students are familiar with other methods. These are of following types:

(a) Berkefeld Filter

It consists of a cylinder made of infusorial earth (kieselguhr). It does not require any pressure and filtration of water is rapid. The candle of cylinder can be sterilized by boiling (Fig. 5.5) after every third day.

(b) Pasteur-Chamberland Filter

This has porous tube made of unglazed porcelain. Bacteria are retained within the tube by mechanical action. This filter is quite effective in freeing the water from all sorts of bacteria. Tobies can be cleaned by brushing with hot water and then sterilization by boiling water (Fig. 5.6).

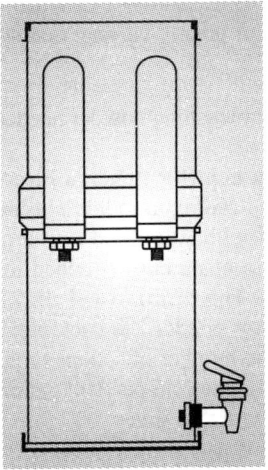
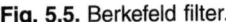

Fig. 5.5. Berkefeld filter.

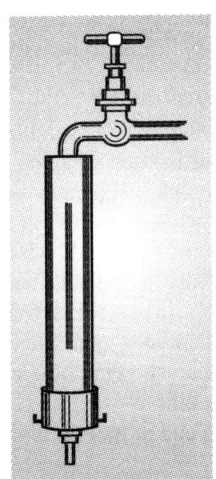

Fig. 5.6. Pasteur-Chamberland filter.

E. Chemicals Used for Water Purification

Alum: It is used in the concentration of 5 to 25 mg/liter of water. Alum reacts with calcium chloride present in water and forms calcium sulfide and aluminum hydrate, which take along the suspended impurities and bacteria present in water at the bottom.

Copper sulfate: In concentration of 0.25 ppm it effectively checks the growth of algae.

Quick lime: It is commonly used for purification of wells and tanks.

Chlorine: *see above.* Chlorine tablets are also available in the market and are used to treat water for drinking and bathing purposes.

Bromine: Used in doses of 3.5 mg/liter of water.

Iodine: Used in concentration of 2 ppm.

Potassium permanganate: It is used in concentration of 0.5 ppm to disinfect wells. It is an effective oxidizing agent.

Nesfield Tablet: The tablet contains iodine, sodium iodide and citric acid. One tablet of 120 mg kills typhoid and cholera organisms in 18 liters of water.

AIR AND VENTILATION

Air is absolutely essential for life. An unlimited relatively clean air is necessary for comfortable and healthy living. While air performs many useful functions like supplying oxygen, respiration, regulation of body temperature etc, polluted air spreads various diseases and their agents. Rapid industrialization and inadequate sanitation are the chief factors in polluting air.

The average composition of air is as follows: Oxygen – 20.95%, Nitrogen – 78 to 79%, Carbon dioxide – 0.03 to 0.04%, Water vapours and ammonia – % varies with temperature; Argon, Neon, Krypton, Helium, and bacteria, spores etc – traces.

The term **air pollution** is applicable when there is an excessive concentration of foreign matter in the outdoor atmosphere, which is harmful to man or his environment. Truly speaking, there is no pure air and hence air pollution is a serious health hazard throughout the world. In India, Delhi is supposed to be the most polluted city in terms of dust concentration in air.

(a) Chief impurities in air

1. Respiration products, mainly CO_2.
2. Dust, fumes, mist, vapours.
3. Harmful gases from industrial sources.
4. Decomposed organic matter giving off ammonia and H_2S with offensive odour.
5. Pollution from natural sources e.g. bacteria, moulds, fungi, and pollens.

(b) Sources of air pollution

1. Process of respiration in men and animals.
2. Automobile combustion and incomplete fuel combustion giving off CO_2, gasoline, oxide etc in big cities.
3. Industrial and other commercial processes dealing with combustion process in cities.
4. Domestic fuel burning.
5. Decomposed organic matter from refuse and dead vegetation.
6. Pollution from natural sources e.g. dust, pollen, bacteria and fungi.

7. Insecticide and pesticide sprays used in agriculture.
8. Radioactive material disposal.

(c) Hazards of polluted air
1. Adverse effects on respiratory system.
2. Increase in morbidity and mortality.
3. Chronic bronchitis and carcinoma of lungs.
4. Reduction of atmospheric visibility.
5. Adverse effects on animal and plant life in long run.
6. General ill effects like headache, giddiness, depression, loss of appetite and lassitude.

Purification of air in natural course also occurs because:
- The wind dilutes, sweeps away or aspirates the impurities and gets replaced by pure air.
- The rain washes the air and removes gases and suspended impurities.
- Oxygen and ozone oxidize the organic matter present in the air.
- Plants absorb CO_2 and give off oxygen in sunlight.
- Sun affects the temperature, pressure and volume of air.
- Changing weather and other climatic and meteorological factors affect the direction and velocity of air movements over vast areas.

(d) General indicators of air pollution
These are helpful in assessing the extent of pollution. These are:
1. Estimate of suspended particles in air (μg/cu m of air).
2. Smoke index, expressed as *coh units*/1000 linear feet of air sample filtered through a standard paper tape and its density recorded with photoelectrometer.
3. Amount of CO_2 formed from fuel, coal, CO, NO_2, lead and other oxides.

In pharmaceutical industry clean air, free from particles and bacteria is obtained by the use of HEPA (High Efficiency Particulate Air) filters and Laminar Flow Stations. This is absolutely essential in the production areas for parenteral preparations.

The National Environmental Engineering Research Institute (NEERI) at Nagpur has been established by WHO as regional centre for monitoring and study of air pollution. Similar laboratories are also established at Mumbai, Delhi, Kolkata, Chennai, Hyderabad, Kanpur, Jaipur and Ahmedabad.

A. Prevention and Control

Air pollution has global significance due to serious health effects, both immediate and long term. For prevention and control of air pollution WHO has recommended the following measures-

1. Containment
It means prevention of escape of toxic polluants into the air by use of engineering methods such as enclosure, ventilation and air cleaning. *Arrestors* have been developed to remove the contaminants from the air.

2. Replacement

It means replacing a process contributing to air pollution by a non-polluting process e.g. using electricity in place of coal or natural gas.

3. Dilution

The method has limited application particularly when excessive pollution takes place. Winds dilute as well as sweep away the impurities in air. Vegetation also removes air polluants. Developing *green belts* between industrial and residential areas is also effective in diluting the air pollution.

4. Legislation

Enactment and strict enforcement of Air Control legislation is the need of the day. The Smoke Nuisance Act is effective in Kolkata, Mumbai, Ahmedabad and Kanpur.

5. International action

The WHO has established an international network of laboratories for the monitoring centres at London, and Washington; 3 regional centers at Moscow, Nagpur and Tokyo; and 20 laboratories in various parts of the world. These centres would issue warnings of air pollution whenever necessary.

AIR DISINFECTION

Disinfection of air is most important in hospital wards and operation theatres where the atmosphere must be maintained free from any infectious microorganisms. It can be achieved by:

1. Mechanical ventilation: This reduces vitiated (contaminated) air and bacterial density.
2. UV radiation: UV lamps are also useful in operation theatres and infectious diseases wards.
3. Chemical means: TEG (triethylene glycol) vapours are effective in killing bacteria in air, particularly in droplet nuclei and dust.
4. Dust control: Oil applied to floors in hospital wards is effective in reducing bacterial content of the air.

VENTILATION

It is a science of maintaining atmospheric conditions, which are comfortable and helpful to the human body. It includes air, temperature and humidity. The major objective of ventilation is to ensure supply of clean, pure air at adequate temperature, humidity and air movements comfortable to the body. This means that the polluted air should be constantly removed and replaced with fresh air to ensure an environment that is comfortable and free from infection hazards.

Inadequate ventilation and overcrowding in rooms causes air pollution due to CO_2 increase, elevated temperature, increased humidity and stagnation.

Internal ventilation is the ventilation of environments like streets and road ensured by wide straight streets, detached house, open spaces and parks in thickly populated areas.

Systems of Ventilation

A. Natural ventilation

It is effective, cheap and satisfactory for small dwellings, schools and offices. The system is based on:

1. Wind: The blowing movement of the air through rooms when doors and windows are open is called *perflation*. It bypasses any obstruction and exerts a suction action at its tail, called *aspiration*. *Cross ventilation* is produced through doors and windows facing each other.
2. Diffusion: According to Graham's Law gases diffuse in inverse proportion to the square root of their densities. Therefore gaseous impurities mix with fresh air and reduce pollution. This process is very slow.
3. Unequal Temperature: Air at high temperature expands and rises up and is replaced by fresh cold air. This is more practical in cold climate. Proper location of windows, doors, ventilators and skylights is necessary for the efficiency of natural ventilation.

B. Artificial ventilation

This system is mostly employed in crowded places like theatres, factories, public halls etc. Three systems are used in practice:

1. Vacuum system: It consists of mechanical suction or extraction of vitiated and foul air.
2. Plenum system: This is a good system. Fresh air is forced into the room by revolving fans or blowers.
3. Balanced system: This is the most satisfactory system. Noise is a combination of vacuum and plenum systems. It forms the basis of air-conditioning.

NOISE

Noise has become a very important 'stress factor' in our environment. It is a nuisance, an unwanted sound that is unpleasant to ears. **Noise pollution** is increasing due to industrialization, heavy machines, technology, transport vehicles, ceremonies, festivals, religious and political activities etc. Unit of measurement of sound and noise is *decibel* (db). A decibel is the smallest difference in sound audible to the ears normally. At 100–120 db noise is uncomfortable and at 130–140 db it is painful to ears. The general noise level should not exceed 85 db. Continued loud noises above 80–90 db may lead to loss of hearing. Audiometer is used to measure hearing ability.

Most common **ill-effects of noise pollution** include (i) general inefficiency resulting in lowered output, (ii) exaggeration of peptic ulcer and cardiovascular diseases, (iii) irritability, nervous tension and neurosis, (vi) physical and mental fatigue with loss of concentration, and (vii) developmental anomalies in fetus etc.

Prevention and Control

Following measures can minimize noise pollution:

1. Use of silencing devices at source.
2. Use of sound absorbing material in machinery.
3. Use of ear plugs or ear muffs by the workers in factories with more than 100 db noise.
4. Banning of musical horns and increasing the *no horn* or *silence zones* for vehicles.
5. Use of loud speakers is the commonest noise measure that should be restricted.
6. Road side houses should have sound proof walls.
7. Heavy vehicular traffic in residential areas should not be permitted.
8. Development of residential areas around loud noise factories should be discouraged.
9. Plantation of trees can help reduce noise by 8-10 db.
10. Educating the general public about the importance of noise as a community hazard.
11. Legislative control.

LIGHT

Light is essential for vision and good lighting is essential for efficient vision.

Requirements of good lighting

The illumination should be good, adequate, constant and uniform. Glare should be avoided, bright light shadows eliminated and there should be no flicker or variation. For certain types of fine work shadow less lighting is essential. Compact Fluorescent Lighting (CFL) should be preferred as it is economical (consumes less electricity), avoids shadows and contrasts and increases the efficiency of workers.

Bad lighting causes eye strain, headache, tendency of deformity such as wry neck, round shoulders, poking head and lateral deviation of spine, irritability, liability to accidents, slovenly habits and lack of tidiness and reduced efficiency.

Lighting could be either natural or artificial.

(i) Natural lighting: It is preferred for reasons of economy and its beneficial effect on health. It is most easily provided by windows, which should have an area of at least one tenth of floor space, but truly speaking window area should be related to the intended purpose of the room.

(ii) Artificial lighting: It should provide adequate, consistent and uniform illumination without flickering or glare and completely devoid of shadows. Artificial light should be as close to daylight as possible in composition. Artificial light can be obtained through candles, paraffin lamps and coal gas but the most important is the electric lighting. Filament lamps are most popular in which the electricity heats up the tungsten filament of the electric bulbs. Fluorescent lamps consist of a glass tube fitted with mercury vapours and an electrode fitted at each end. Fluorescent chemicals coat the inside surface of the tube and absorb practically all the UV radiation and remit the radiation in visible range. They are cool and efficient and emit the light, which is just like natural light.

Indirect electric light is the best especially when reflected from the ceiling.

SOLID WASTE DISPOSAL AND CONTROL

- *Waste* is the solid and liquid matter form household and environments, and includes commercial and industrial wastes.
- *Solid waste* is also called refuse in cities and litter in villages. It consists of garbage, ashes and all rubbish discarded from houses and environments except human excreta.
- *Liquid waste* is from humans and animals, laundry, kitchen, street, commercial and industrial wastes.

Waste becomes a source of spread of pathogens and diseases like enteric fever, cholera, bacillary dysentery and amoebic dysentery, infectious hepatitis, helminthic infections etc are transmitted through human waste. Waste disposal is therefore important from public health viewpoint. The objective is to protect health, preserve our natural resources, maintain healthy environment and prevent nuisance conditions.

(a) Sources of refuse

- *Household refuse* includes food waste, dust, ashes, rugs, papers, animal droppings etc. Affluent societies in general produce more and more bulk refuse.
- *Street refuse* includes dust, dung, paper, bird droppings, animal and vegetable wastes and other droppings.
- *Industrial refuse* consists of a wide variety of wastes ranging from inert material like calcium carbonate to highly toxic and explosive compounds.
- *Stable refuse* is collected from stables and contains waste straw, dust, dung etc.
- *Domestic refuse* consists of ash, rubbish and garbage. Rubbish comprises of paper, clothing bits of wood, metal, glass, dust and dirt.
- *Garbage* is the waste matter resulting from preparation, cooking and consumption of foods and consists of waste food, vegetable peelings and other organic matter. Garbage ferments on storage hence it must be quickly disposed.

(b) Collection and removal of refuse

Sanitary bins should be used for collection of household refuse to avoid putrefaction and fly breeding. Street refuse is collected by conservancy staff. It should be kept in specially provided public bins. The refuse so collected should be transported to places of disposal in covered carts or motor vans etc.

(c) Disposal of refuse

Following methods are commonly used for disposal of refuse:

1. Controlled tipping and dumping

Controlled tipping is an easy and cheap method. The refuse is generally utilized in filling up clay pits and hollows, in sanitary tanks or in reclaiming low lying lands. Indiscriminate dumping causes nuisance from fire, flies, rats and offensive gases. Dumping sites should be 30–50 metres away from habitation. Refuse material should be deposited in layers of about 6′ and covered with about 9″ thick layer of earth. According to WHO, dumping is a most unsanitary method that creates public health hazards and leads to pollution of environment.

2. Burning or incineration

It is one of the best methods of refuse disposal. Burning makes the refuse harmless and reduces it to $1/4^{th}$ of its original weight. The mass left behind is hard clinker, which is used in making roads. The incineration is carried out in a furnace constructed of bricks with firebrick lining.

3. Composting

This method is useful in towns where refuse has to be disposed off with night soil and converted into compost, which has high manure value. Composting is a process of changing organic matter into manure with the help of bacterial action. Excreta, refuse and moisture are mixed in a suitable proportion to give carbon : nitrogen ratio of 30 : 1. Two-week-old inoculum of bacteria is also added. The mixture is laid in dug out trenches (3′ deep and 6–8′ wide with adjustable length till the layer is 6″ to 9″ above ground level). Then it is covered with earth. Composting is completed in 4 to 6 months time.

4. Mechanical composting

This is a development in composting, which is currently practiced in Holland, Germany, Switzerland and Israel. Mechanical composting plants are likely to be set up by the Government of India in cities with over 5-lakh population. The process consists of first removing salvable materials such as rags, bones, metal, glass etc from refuse. It is then pulverized to reduce the size of the particles to less than 2″. The pulverized refuse is mixed with nightsoil, sewage or sludge in a rotating machine and incubated. The compost gets ready in 4 to 6 weeks time.

5. Pitting

This method is particularly useful in rural areas. The refuse is dumped into manure pits and covered with earth. In about 6 months the refuse is converted into valuable manure.

6. Burial

In this method refuse is buried into an excavated trench of 1.5 meter width and 2 meter depth and covered with 20 to 30 cm of earth at the end of each day.

When the level of dumped material in the trench comes to 40 cm above the ground level, the trench is filled with earth and composted and a new trench excavated.

7. Disposal in sea

Refuse at airports can be dumped in deep sea, at least 8 to 10 Km away from seashore. This is an expensive method.

Public education about the importance of refuse disposal would go a long way in solving the problem. The International Solid Wastes and Public Cleansing Association assists various countries in the general endeavor to improve sanitary services. Information about waste disposal can also be obtained from WHO International Reference Centre in Switzerland.

EXCRETA DISPOSAL

Human excreta are a potential source of infection and pollution. Improper excreta disposal may (i) pose health hazards like soil pollution, water pollution, contamination of foods and propagation of flies; (ii) cause diseases like typhoid and paratyphoid, fever, dysentery, diarrhoeas, cholera, hookworm infestation, and parasitic infestations. The problem is more serious in India where only 15% of the urban population has the amenity of a sewerage system. Most of the population lives in rural areas and defecates in fields. This pollutes the environment. It is estimated that about 5 million people in India die every year due to intestinal group of diseases.

Thus proper disposal of human excreta constitutes a fundamental environmental health service.

The infectious organisms present in the human excreta of sick persons act as disease carrier and constitute the chief source of infection. Transmission of infectious organisms into susceptible host from excreta may take place through water, soil, fingers, flies and food (Fig. 5.7A). The cycle is best interrupted at the level of source i.e. excreta. Thus proper disposal of excreta is the most important method, which can offer a **sanitation barrier** as shown in Fig. 5.7B. Sanitation barrier could be a sanitary latrine or a sanitary pit.

Methods of excreta disposal

There are two main systems of excreta disposal:

(a) Conservancy system

The principle of this system is that filth, refuse and all other putrefiable matters should not be exposed to flies, should not contaminate the water and should be transported for safe disposal. Excreta are removed by manual labor from privies and latrines.

Privy means structure for depositing excreta in private houses while *latrines* are similar structures for public use.

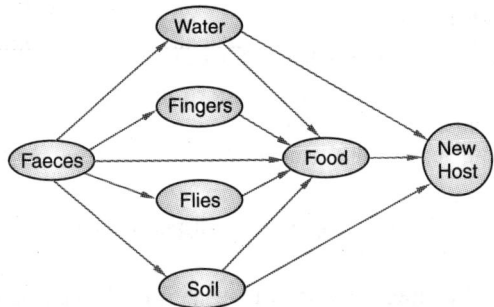

Fig. 5.7A. Transmission of infection through faeces.

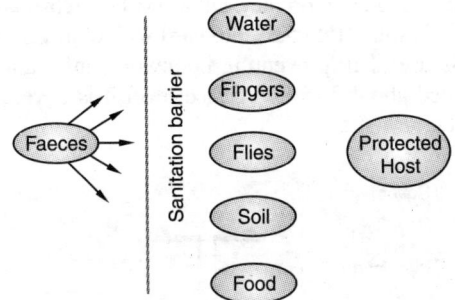

Fig. 5.7 B. Sanitation barrier for transmission of infection through faeces.

TYPE OF PRIVIES AND LATRINES

Privy system: Privy is meant for private use hence it should be constructed at the ground floor of the house at a distance of 6' from living room and about 40' from the nearest well or source of water supply. It consists of a chamber made of bricks with cement lining and provided with a proper seat. A small window for ventilation and air supply should also be provided. Although privy system is simplest yet most unsanitary. There remains the possibility of leakage and pollution of water and soil. Besides, buckets and pan get corroded and require replacement.

Pail system: Here a receptacle is placed under the squatting seat and excreta removed into pail carts for disposal.

Commode: This system is more popular in urban areas at places where there is no adequate water carriage system. It consists of wooden or plastic seat with self-closing lid and enamel pot to receive excreta. The sweeper empties the pail from the commode after use, which is then cleaned and refitted.

The privy, pail and commode types are also know as **service types** but these should be replaced by sanitary latrines, which don't require service and excreta can be disposed of in a hygienic manner.

Sanitary latrines

The requirements of a sanitary latrine are as follows:

• The excreta is not accessible to carriers of infection like flies, rodents, and animals e.g. pigs, dogs, cattle etc.

• Excreta do not create a nuisance due to offensive smell or unsightly appearance.

Sanitary latrines are most important for disposal of human excreta. Common types are described below:

Bored Hole Latrine: This type of latrine is recommended for rural areas. It was introduced in 1930 by the Rockfeller Foundation. It consists of a circular hole (14 to 16″ diameter) penetrating 18 to 20′ into ground water. It should reach subsoil water 3′ in depth. The opening is covered with squatting plate and superstructure is made for privacy. Dilution of excreta takes place in subsoil water. The latrine is sunk (Fig. 5.8) into hard soil to prevent its collapse. This type of latrine is useful in preventing hookworm infestation in rural areas. When hole is filled about 3′ from surface level it is covered with earth and another is dug at a new site.

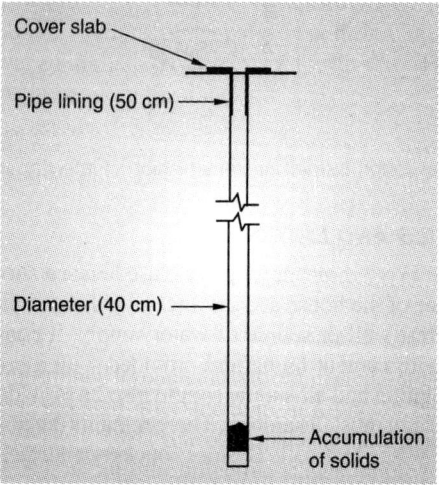

Fig. 5.8. Bored hole latrine.

Dug Well Latrine: This type is also recommended for rural areas. It consists of a 15 to 20′ deep pit with 3′ diameter. It is provided with ½″ water seal and a squatting plate of 3.5′ diameter. It can be flushed with 3 liters of water. Water seal prevents flies and offensive smell. When filled up to about 3′ from surface level they are filled with earth and new one dug at a new site. The construction is economical and excreta are quickly disposed off with septic tank like action. Dug well latrine is better than bored hole latrine.

Two more important types of latrines are (i) PRAI type evolved by the Planning, Research and Action Institute, Lucknow; and (ii) the RCA evolved by the Research-Cum-Action Projects in Environmental Sanitation of the Ministry of Health, Government of India. Both are similar except in minor engineering details.

RCA Latrine: Selection of site – Site should be selected inside a house and at a distance of 15 metres from the nearest source of water supply and should be at a lower elevation to prevent possibility of bacterial contamination of water supply.

Squatting plate: Minimum dimensions of squatting plate (Fig. 5.9) are 90 cm × 90 cm × 5 cm. It is made of impervious material like glazed stone, cement or concrete for ease of washing and keeping clean and dry. Circular squatting plates (90 cm diameter, 5 cm thickness) are also used. A 1/2″ slope towards the pan is also provided so that the water used for cleansing purposes (ablution) may drain out. Rigid footrests over the plate are provided for convenience of the user so that they ease out comfortably, in appropriate position.

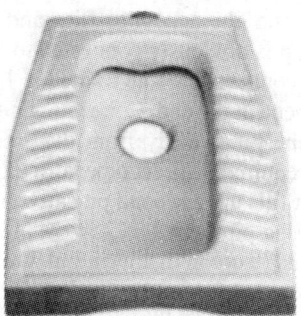

Fig. 5.9. Squatting plate.

Pan: All the night soil, urine and wash water are received in the latrine pan. It measures 42.5 cm in length but varies from front portion (12.5 cm) to widest portion (20 cm) (Fig. 5.10). A uniform slope from front to back allows drainage of the material. The pan should have smooth finish for good washing and cleaning etc.

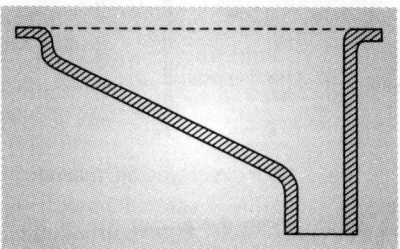

Fig. 5.10. Pan.

Trap: A trap consists of a pipe (7.5 cm diameter), bent upon itself in such a way that it retains certain amount of water in the bend. The purpose of using a trap is to hold water and provide necessary *water seal* i.e. the distance between the level of water in the trap at the lowest point in the concave upper surface of the trap (Fig. 5.11).

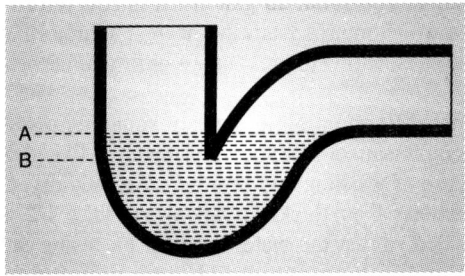

Fig. 5.11. Trap.

The water seal prevents the access to flies and suppresses the nuisance from foul smell. The trap is obviously connected to the pan.

Connecting pipe: It connects the trap to the pit. It is 1 metre long with 7.5 cm diameter and has a bend at the end. Connecting pipe is used in indirect type RCA latrine because the pit is away from the squatting plate (Fig. 5.12). Connecting pipe is not required in direct type latrine. The advantage of indirect pipe is that when the pit fills up, a second pit can be used just by changing the direction of the connecting pipe.

The pit or dug well is 75 cm in diameter and 3 to 3.5 metre deep.

Superstructure is provided for privacy and shelter.

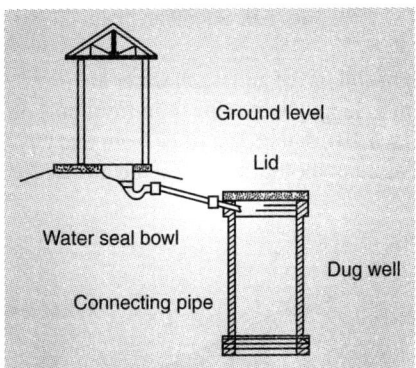

Fig. 5.12. Indirect type RCA latrine.

Education of the public about the proper use of RCA latrine is essential. Pan must be flushed after use with 1.5 liters of water. The squatting plate should not be soiled. Latrine should not be used for dumping of refuse or other debris.

Septic Tanks: Septic tanks (Fig. 5.13) were first introduced in 1906 for the disposal of liquid waste and excreta but not connected to public sewerage system. Anaerobic digestion of solid waste in the subsoil outside the tank brings about purification of sewage. Length of the chamber is twice its breadth and it is 1.5 to 2 metre deep. Inlet and outlet pipes are submerged. The capacity of household tanks should be about 25 gallons. It is covered by a concrete slab and provided with a manhole for inspection.

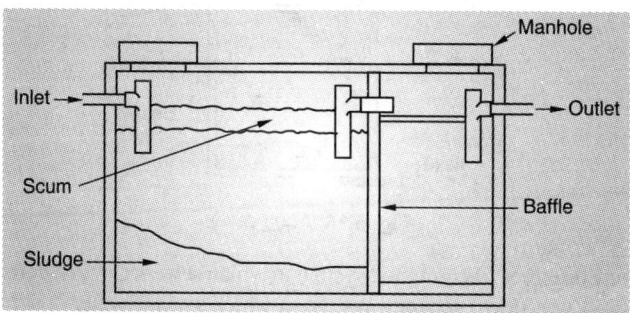

Fig. 5.13. Septic tank.

Because the purification of sewage in septic tank depends on the bacterial flora, use of soap water and disinfectants should be avoided. The contents of the septic tank should be emptied out at least once a year (dislodging).

Sulabh Sauchalaya: *Sulabh sauchalaya* is an improved version of RCA type latrine. It is a low cost, pour-flush, water seal type of latrine. The method requires very little water and excreta undergo bacterial decomposition. Sulabh International also maintains community latrines. Such latrines have been constructed in many cities throughout India even at railway stations and bus stands.

Trench latrines: These are simple dug trenches recommended for temporary use in fairs, military camps etc and may be either shallow or deep type.

Aqua Privy: It is a small septic tank like system. Excreta go into a tank where septic action takes place. Tank is ventilated by a pipe opening in outside air. Effluent from tank flows into garden or soak pit (Fig. 5.14). It could be rectangular or circular in shape. Size of aqua privy can be varied for use to individual families or general public.

(b) Water Carriage System (Sewerage System)

Sewage includes excreta, urine, house water and rain water along with water from stables, factories etc. Water carriage system comprises of collecting human excreta, urine, water and waste from residential, industrial and commercial areas by a flush of water through a network of underground pipes (sewers) and transporting to far off place outside the town. This is the most sanitary method if plenty of water is available. It is also called sewage or **sewerage system,**

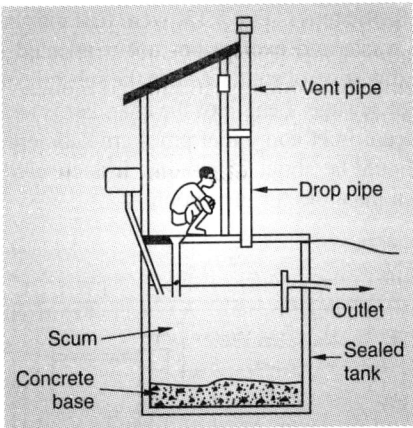

Fig. 5.14. Aqua privy.

which may be either (i) combined system in which sewers carry both the sewage and storm water, or (ii) separate system in which surface water is not admitted into sewers.

Essential requirements for the successful working of water carriage system are:
1. Abundant water supply for flushing water closet.
2. Good underground drains and sewers with proper ventilation.
3. Sufficient fall to give required velocity to the sewage.
4. Proper methods of utilization of sewage.

Essential elements of a water carriage system are discussed below:

1. *Household sanitary fittings:* These include water closet, urinal and wash basin. Water closet is a sanitary installation for reception of excreta and is connected with sewer through soil pipe and house drain. It works by siphon action and consists of a basin and a trap (closet proper) and flushing apparatus (cistern) having 15 litres capacity, connected with closet type pipe. An ideal water closet is shown in Fig. 5.15.

2. *House drain:* Water closet is connected to house drain through soil pipe. The soil pipe is made of cast iron with internal diameter of 10 cm and extending 1 to 1.5 metres above the roof for escape of offensive gases from house drain. It should be situated outside the house.

House drain is the underground pipe connecting soil pipe with sewer and empties the sewage into the main sewer or public drain.

3. *Public sewer:* Sewage from several houses is collected through trunk sewers and transported to the place of final disposal. Trunk sewers may be small (not less than 9″) or bigger (2 to 3 metres) laid on a bed of cement concrete, about 3 metres below the ground level.

Manholes provided in the sewerage system permit inspection, repair and cleaning. Traps are also provided to prevent foul gases entering the houses and to remove sand, grit and grease form sewage.

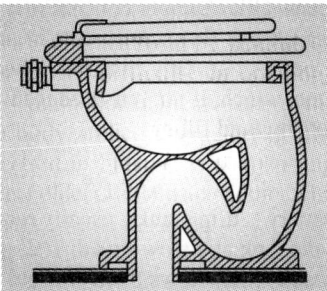

Fig. 5.15. Water closet system.

DISPOSAL OF SEWAGE

The main purpose of disposal of sewage is to convert different unstable organic matters present in sewage into harmless stable chemical compounds. Sewage generally contains 99.9% water plus organic and inorganic impurities. But it is the organic matter, which imparts offensive nature to the sewage. Either aerobic or anaerobic processes bring about decomposition of organic matter. In aerobic process the organic matter is broken down into simpler compounds like carbon dioxide, water, ammonia, nitrites, nitrates and sulphates by the action of bacteria, fungi and protozoa. The end products of anaerobic process are methane, ammonia, carbon dioxide and hydrogen.

The disposal of sewage into water course may be carried out *(i)* by dilution (without prior treatment), or *(ii)* by purification (after prior treatment).

1. By Dilution

The method consists of diluting sewerage by discharging it into sea or river water. It can be applied in places near sea or the riverside. It must be ensured that the dilution is sufficient. Disposal of sewage into rivers makes the water polluted and unsafe for potable purposes.

The best method of sewage disposal is therefore disposal after purification. The objective is to collect, treat and dispose off sewage in such a manner that will protect health, preserve our natural resources and prevent nuisance factors and water-borne diseases.

2. By Purification

Purification is done through either preliminary or secondary treatment.

Preliminary treatment

It removes solids by passing through screens and grit chambers. Bar screens remove gross solids like stones, bricks, dead animals etc. The screen consists of iron bars 2.5 to 4 cm apart and set at 33 to 60º angles in direction of sewage flow. Comminutor may be used in place of screens. **Comminutor** is a mechanical grinder, which crushes larger solids to smaller size that can pass through 1 cm apart screens. Grit chamber consists of a long, narrow and deep channel. In this chamber sewage flows at the rate of one foot per second, the grit settles and sewage passes out. Grit consists of heavy inorganic material like sand, gravel, glass etc, which, if not removed, causes wear and tear of the plant. Grit is disposed off by land filling.

Primary treatment

This is carried out in primary settling tanks, usually rectangular in design. The sewage passes through the tank at a slow speed, 1–2′ per minute and remains in the tank for 6 to 8 hours. This allows solids to settle to form sludge at the bottom followed by removal by sludge collectors. The scum rises at the top and removed into a scum-removing trough near the outlet.

Pre-treatment removes about 50% of solids and suspended matter and reduces the coliform bacteria by 30 to 40%. The Biological Oxygen Demand (BOD) of sewage is reduced by about one third. *BOD* is the amount of oxygen needed to oxidize organic matter in the sewage.

Secondary treatment

This is carried either by trickling filter unit or activated sludge unit. Biological action takes place and organic matter in the sewage is converted into inorganic nitrates by aerobic bacteria. This reduces BOD of sewage by about 90%.

Trickling Filter Unit: After primary treatment, the sewage effluent is led to trickling filters, which consist of a bed of crushed stones or clinker, 6–100′ in diameter and 5–6′ deep. During the passage through filters, the bacterial flora oxidizes the effluent. The sewage is then taken to secondary settling tanks for the settlement of sludge. The resulting effluent is treated with chlorine and discharged into a river or a stream.

Activated Sludge Unit: Activated sludge process is also known as *biaeration process*. It is aerobic process of disposal of sewage and is considered to be most satisfactory method of sewage purification. The sewage effluent is mixed (Fig. 5.16) with 15 to 25% of activated sludge from the secondary settling tanks, mixed with compressed air and left in aeration tank for 4 to 8 hours for the biological action. The organic matter in the sewage is thus converted into stable inorganic form. The typhoid and cholera organisms are destroyed and coliforms are greatly reduced.

The sewage effluent after preliminary treatment and primary treatment is carried to the mixing chambers of aeration chambers in which whole of sewage are converted into fine emulsion with the help of compressed air. The scum is removed from top and sewage led to mixing chambers. In mixing chamber the sewage is mixed with 15 to 25% of activated sludge obtained from secondary settling tanks. The mixed sewage is then led to aeration tanks where it is agitated by compressed air through diffusers. The aeration period is 4 to 8 hours. The organic matter breaks up and ammonia is oxidized to nitrates. Sewage from aeration tanks flows to secondary settling tanks where coagulated material settles and forms activated sludge. A portion of this activated sludge is again

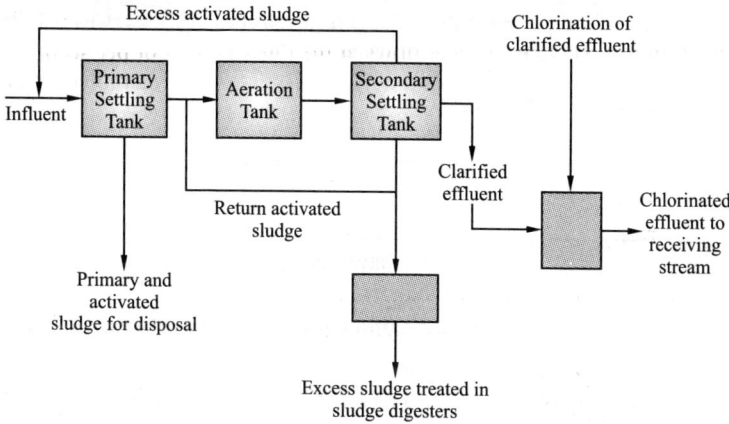

Fig. 5.16. Activated sludge unit.

used for mixing with sewage in mixing chambers and remaining portion is taken for process of digestion.

The effluent from secondary settling tanks may be chlorinated to destroy pathogenic organisms and finally discharged to water course.

Sludge digestion is the process of sludge fermentation under anaerobic conditions. This digestion produces (i) inofffensive sludge, much reduced in amount and easily handled, and (ii) burnable gas.

A modern sewage treatment plant is shown in Fig. 5.17.

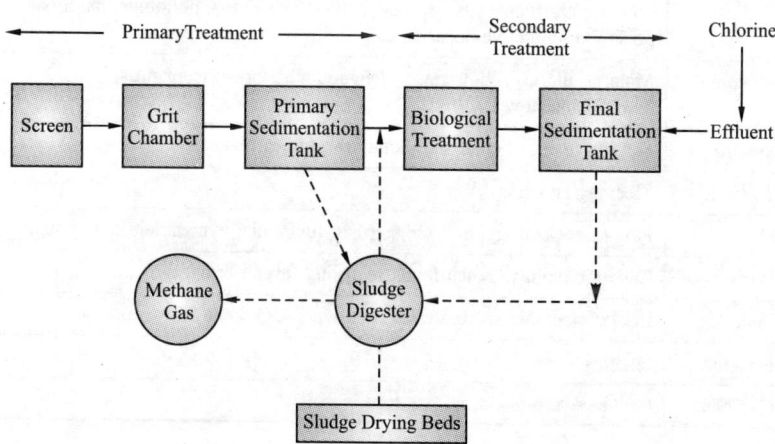

Fig. 5.17. Modern sewage treatment plant.

MEDICAL ENTOMOLOGY

Medical entomology means the study of the arthropods of medical importance. It is an important branch of preventive medicine. Arthropods occur in the environment around us. Besides destroying the crops and food reserves, they act as carriers or vectors of many diseases.

Classification of Arthropods

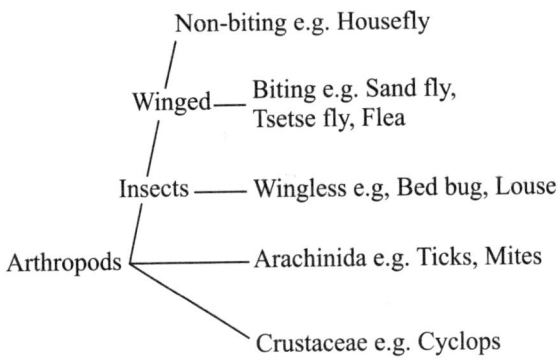

Diseases caused by common arthropods

These are given in Table 5.2.

Arthropod	Diseases Transmitted
Housefly	Cholera, diarrhoeas, amoebic dysentery, enteric fever, tuberculosis, typhoid, gastroenteritis, leprosy, anthrax, trachoma, poliomyelitis, food poisoning, infective hepatitis etc
Mosquito	Malaria, filaria, yellow fever, dengue fever, viral encephalitis, hemorrhagic fever
Sandfly	Sandfly fever, oriental sore, kala-azar, Oraya fever
Tsetse fly	Sleeping sickness
Flea	Plague, endemic typhus, chiggerosis, tularemia, hymenolepsis diminuta
Louse	Endemic typhus, trench fever, relapsing fever, dermatitis
Tick	Rocky mountain spotted fever, tick typhus, Q fever
Itch mite	Scabies
Cyclops	Guinea worm infection, fish tape worm

Table 5.2. Diseases caused by common arthropods

A. Mode of Disease Transmission

Arthropod-borne diseases are transmitted into human beings in the following ways:

1. Direct Contact: Arthropods are transmitted directly from man to man through direct contact e.g. scabies and pediculosis.

2. Mechanical Transmission: It is the mechanical transmission of the disease agent by the arthropod e.g. diarrhoea, dysentery etc.
3. Biological Transmission: In this mode the disease agent multiplies or undergoes some developmental change in the arthropod host e.g. plague, malaria, and filariasis.

B. Control of Arthropods

General measures for the control of arthropods comprise of:

1. Environmental Control: This is the best method. All possible breeding places for insects must be eliminated. Most important aspect is to prevent collection and stagnation of water at any place. Stagnated water is the most common breeding place of arthropods. There should be prompt and safe disposal of human excreta and organic refuse by suitable methods. Supply of safe and potable water to the community must be ensured. It is also necessary to keep the surroundings clean and protect all foods from insects.
2. Chemical Control: It is based on the use of chemicals (insecticides) to eradicate larva and adult insect at breeding places. Commonly used insecticides include DDT (dichlorodiphenyltrichloroethane), BHC (benzene hexachloride), chlordane, malathion, pyrethrum etc.
3. Genetic Control: It is based on restricting the propagation of insects (especially mosquitoes) by techniques such as 'sterile male technique' (breeding sterile males), cytoplasmic incompatibility, replacement of genes etc.
4. Biological Control: It consists of using biological agents for the control of insects e.g. propagation of Gambusia fish to eradicate larvae of mosquito.

However no single method is satisfactory hence use of two or more combined methods is recommended.

C. Common Arthropods

(a) House-fly

House-fly is the most important amongst flies. Its presence indicates unsanitary conditions. It breeds on excreta, cowdung and decomposed matter. The breeding is faster in humid climate. Its average life is about 2 to 4 weeks. Houseflies act as mechanical carriers of disease and carry germs on their body, legs and wings. It also ingests germs and vomits or defecates on food, milk and causes the disease. Life cycle of housefly has four stages: egg, larva, pupa, adult (Fig. 5.18).

Anti-fly measures include prevention of breeding of flies, protection of food from flies, destruction of adult flies, use of poisonous chemicals and insecticidal sprays etc.

(b) Mosquito

Important varieties of mosquitoes in India are *Anopheles* (spreads malaria), *Culex* (causes filariasis and encephalitis), *Mansonia* (cause of yellow fever among monkeys) and *Aedes* (spreads yellow fever, dengue fever, hemorrhogic

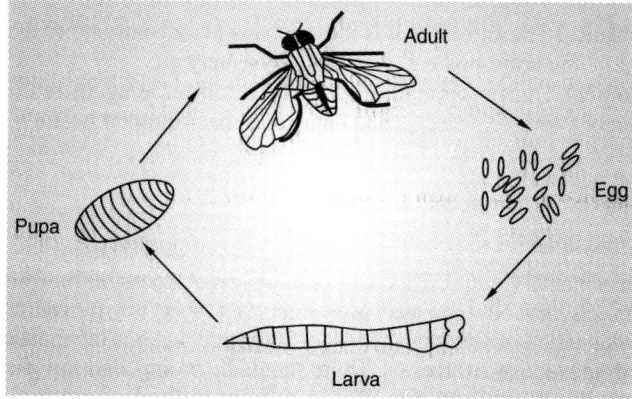

Fig. 5.18. Life cycle of house-fly.

fever). There are four stages in the life history of mosquitoes; egg, larva, pupa and adult (Fig. 5.19). The first three stages are spent in water therefore the presence of water is absolutely essential for their existence.

The male mosquito feeds on vegetables but the female feeds on the blood of the host.

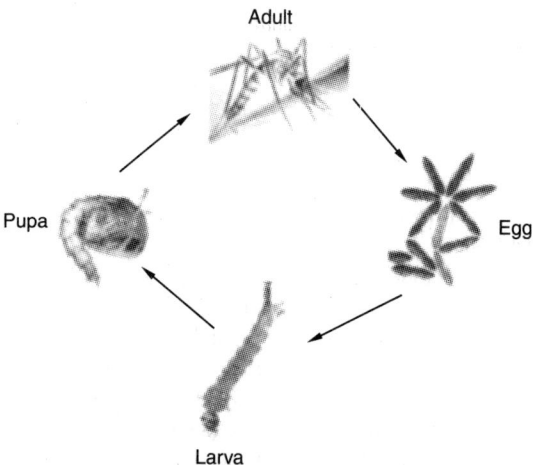

Fig. 5.19. Life cycle of mosquito.

(c) Fleas

They are wingless, 2 to 3 mm long with lateral compressed highly chitinous body. They commonly live in rodents and in the absence of rodents they bite man.

Life cycle: egg-larva-pupa-adult.

Fleas transmit diseases through biting, mechanical transmission and faeces. Most important disease transmitted by fleas in plague.

(d) Lice

They are 2 to 3 mm long, wingless insects having hard chitinous covering with 3 pairs of legs each provided with a single claw. They are ectoparasites mainly of birds. The lice infesting man are of three types.

Pediculus capitis	Head louse	} *Pediculus humanus*
Pediuculus corporis	Body louse	
Plothirus pubis	On pubic hair and eyelashes	

Life cycle: egg-larva-adult.

Infestation is by direct contact, through combs, brushes, clothing etc.

Lice are vectors of epidemic typhus, relapsing fever, trench fever and dermatitis.

(e) Ticks

Ticks are blood suckers found in warm climate. They are ectoparasites of vertebrate animals.

Hard ticks (*Ixodidae*) have a scutum (shield) with mouthparts on dorsal surface. These are attached to the host like lice.

Soft ticks (*Agrasidae*) are without scutum with mouthparts on the ventral surface. These feed and leave the host like bed bugs.

Hard ticks transmit Rocky Mountain spotted fever, viral encephalitis, viral fever etc. Soft ticks transmit Q fever, relapsing fever etc. Diseases are transmitted by bites.

(f) Cyclops (Water flea)

It is a crustacean mostly present in fresh water. It swims in water with characteristic jerky movements. The average life of a cyclops is about 3 months. It acts as an intermediate host of guinea worm disease.

(g) Rodents

Rodents are very common in man's environment. They are not only a health hazards but also cause damage to buildings, foodstuffs and other commodities. Most important domestic rodents are black rat (*Rattus rattus*), Norway rat or sewer rat (*R. Norvegians*) and the house rat (*Muss musculus*).

Diseases transmitted through rodents are bacterial (plague, tularemia, salmonellosis; viral (Lassa fever, hemorrhogic fever, encephalitis); rickettsial (scrub typhus, murine typhus, rickettsial pox); others (rat bite, fever, leptospirosis, ringworm etc). These diseases may be transmitted directly through rat bite or through contamination of food, water or through rat fleas.

Anti-rodent measures include sound environmental sanitation, trapping of rats and use of rodenticides like barium carbonate, zinc phosphide, fumigation with calcium cyanide (cynogen), carbon disulfide, methyl bromide, sulfur dioxide etc.

Animals

Animals are most closely associated with human life. More than 150 diseases in man are transmitted through animals. These are termed **zoonoses**. Zoonotic diseases can be due to viruses, bacteria, rickettsiae, fungi, helminths, protozoa, arthropods or insects. Zoonotic infections occurring commonly in India are brucellosis, rabies, tuberculosis, leptospirosis, and hydatid disease.

6

Fundamental Principles of Microbiology

INTRODUCTION

Microorganisms or microbes are living organisms, which are so small that they can't be seen without the use of microscope. **Microbiology** deals with the study of microorganisms while medical microbiology deals with the study of those microorganisms which cause infectious diseases as well the methods of protection against such diseases.

History of Microbiology

Use of magnifying glasses and development of microscopes was the most important landmark in the history of microbiology. In the 1660's **Robert Hooke** used a compound microscope with a magnification of 200 X and studied moulds. **Antoni van Leeuwenhoek**, a Dutch investigator made a detailed study of bacteria, protozoa etc in 1683 using his microscopes with a magnification of 300 X. Since then a variety of microscopes have been developed that can magnify any object by several thousand times.

The ancient people believed in **spontaneous generation** (*abiogenesis*) i.e. they believed that creatures like frogs, mice, bees and other animals sprang from fertile mud, warm rain, fog etc. But scientists all over the world carried scientific experiments during 17th to 19th centuries and ultimately proved that the theory of *abiogenesis* was wrong and the theory of *biogenesis* (life comes from life) was right.

Edward Jenner of England developed vaccine against *smallpox* in 1798. **Jenner** and **Pasteur** gave the principle of active immunization. **Louis Pasteur** (1822-1895), a French scientist made a detailed study of fermentation in the manufacture of beer and wines. His technique of sterilization of milk (*pasteurization*) is used even today in dairies. Phagocytosis was described in 1884 by **Metchnikoff**, a Russian scientist. A virus causing sarcoma in fowls was isolated in 1911 by **Peyton Rous**. The antibiotic era started with the discovery of penicillin by **Sir Alexender Fleming** in 1929. Prontosil was discovered in 1935 by **Domagk**.

Microorganisms are now employed for various beneficial purposes to human race like vaccination, fermentation, antibiotic production, food industry, dairy industry and even in sewage treatment. Genetic engineering is a new field where improved strains of useful microorganisms are prepared and employed in the production of many products useful to human beings.

CLASSIFICATION OF MICROORGANISMS

Taxonomy is the systematic arrangement of organisms in groups. *Nomenclature* is the science of systematic naming. Microorganisms may have the characteristics of plant as well as animal kingdoms. Because of this difficulty microorganisms were put into a separate kingdom, **Prostista** and hence the simplest classification of microorganisms is as follows.

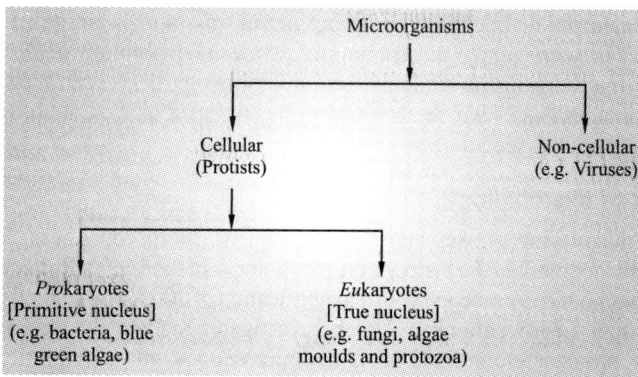

From the view point of a pharmacist, bacteria are the most important microorganism hence the classification of bacteria is being discussed in detail.

Classification of Bacteria

Bacteria can be classified on the basis of different criteria.

1. Oxygen requirements – Aerobic and anaerobic.
2. Energy source – Autotrophs, heterotrophs, phototrophs, chemotrophs.
3. Growth temperature – Thermophilic, mesophilic, psychrophilic.
4. Nutritional requirements – Simple and complex.
5. Ability to grow in living tissues – Saprophytes, parasites, commensals.

(a) Biological classification

It is based on characteristics like physiological, immunological and ecological.

Division: Protophyta
Class: Schizomycetes.
  Orders: Pseudomonadales
      Eubacteriales
      Actinomycetales
      Spirochaetales
      Mycoplasmatales

(b) Morphological classification

It is based on morphological characteristics.

(i) Higher bacteria

These are filamentous and grow by branching to form mycelium.

Actinomycetes –
  (a) Vegetative mycelium fragments into bacillary or cocoid elements.
      (i) Anaerobic, acid-fast, e.g. *Nocardia.*
      (ii) Anaerobic, non-acid-fast, e.g. *Actinomyces bovis.*
  (b) Vegetative mycelium not fragmenting into bacillary or coccoid forms.
      Coccoids are formed in chains from aerial hyphae e.g. *Streptomyces.*

(ii) Lower (true) bacteria

They are unicellular and never from mycelium. They are grouped on the basis of their shape.

(a) Spherical – Cocci
(b) Rod-shaped – Bacilli
(c) Comma-shaped – Vibrio
(d) Spiral – Spirilla
(e) Spirally twisted, flexous rods – Spirochaetes

(c) Numerical classification

It is also called Adansonian classification. It determines the degree of relationship between strains of microbes by a statistical coefficient. Similar and dissimilar characters are given equal importance. Organisms are scored for a number of phenotypic characters. +1 score is given if a character is present and -1 score is given if a character is absent. The degree of similarity of strains A and B is indicated by *similarity index* (S).

$$S = \frac{Ns \text{ (No. of shared or positive characters)}}{Ns \text{ (No. of shared or positive characters)} - Nd \text{ (No. of differences detected)}} \times 100$$

(d) Biochemical classification

Differences in the biochemical components in the structure of prokaryotic or eukaryotic cells, cell membranes etc form the basis of biochemical classification e.g. prokaryotic cell membrane lacks sterols while eukaryotic cells lacks N-acetyl muramic acid.

(e) Genetic classification

Guanine and cytosine (G + C) contents of bacterial composition form the basis of genetic classification. The G + C contents vary greatly in DNA of different bacteria from 25 to 80 mole percent in different genera e.g. G + C in *Clostridium tetani* is 30 to 32% and in *Mycobacterium tuberculosis* it is 60 to 68%. Important differences between prokaryotic and eukaryotic bacteria are shown in Table 6.1.

Table 6.1. Differences between prokaryotic and eukaryotic bacteria

Characteristics	Prokaryote	Eukaryote
1. Nuclear area		
• Nuclear membrane	–	+
• Nucleolus	–	+
• Chromosome number	1	More than 1
• Mitotic division	–	+
2. Cytoplasm		
• Mitochondria	–	+
• Golgi apparatus	–	+
• Lysosomes	–	+
• Cytoplasmic streaming	–	+
• Pinocytosis	–	+
• Endoplasmic reticulum	–	+
3. Chemical composition		
• Sterol	–	+
• Muramic acid	+	–
• Diaminopimelic acid	– or +	–

(+) = present; (–) = absent

BACTERIA

Bacteria are microscopic, rigid walled, unicellular, free-living organisms without chlorophyll, having either DNA or RNA. They are capable of performing all essential functions of life e.g. growth, metabolism and reproduction. They belong to the class Schizomycetes and Order Eubacteriales.

A. Morphological Features of Bacteria

Some important morphological features of bacteria are:

(i) Size

Most of the bacteria are extremely small hence their size is measured in terms of micrometers (μm). Structural details of bacteria and viruses are measured in terms of nanometers (nm) and the minute structural details of cells are expressed in terms of Angstrom (Å).

1 micrometer (μm) or 1 micron (μ) = 1/1000 millimeter
1 nanometer (nm) or 1 millimicron (mμ) = 1/1000 micron
1 Angstrom unit (Å) = 1/10 nanometer

Most spherical bacteria (cocci) are approximately 1 μm in diameter and rod-shaped bacteria (bacilli) are 2 to 10 μm in length and 0.2 to 0.5μm in width.

(ii) Shape and arrangement

Bacteria commonly have following shapes and arrangements.

(a) Coccus – Cocci (from kokkos, meaning berry) are spherical or ellipsoidal.
Cocci in pair – Diplococci e.g. pneumococci, gonococci, meningococci
Cocci in cluster – Staphylococci e.g. *Staphylococcus aureus*
Cocci in chain – Streptococci e.g. *Streptococcus lactis*
Cocci in group of four – Tetrad
Cocci in group of eight – Sarcina

(b) Bacilli are rod-shaped organisms – Rods provide a higher surface area to volume ratio and hence the number of rod shaped bacteria is far greater than that of spherical bacteria. The ends of the bacilli may be square cut, rounded, pointed or from clubs.

(c) Coccobacilli – They are usually short bacilli.

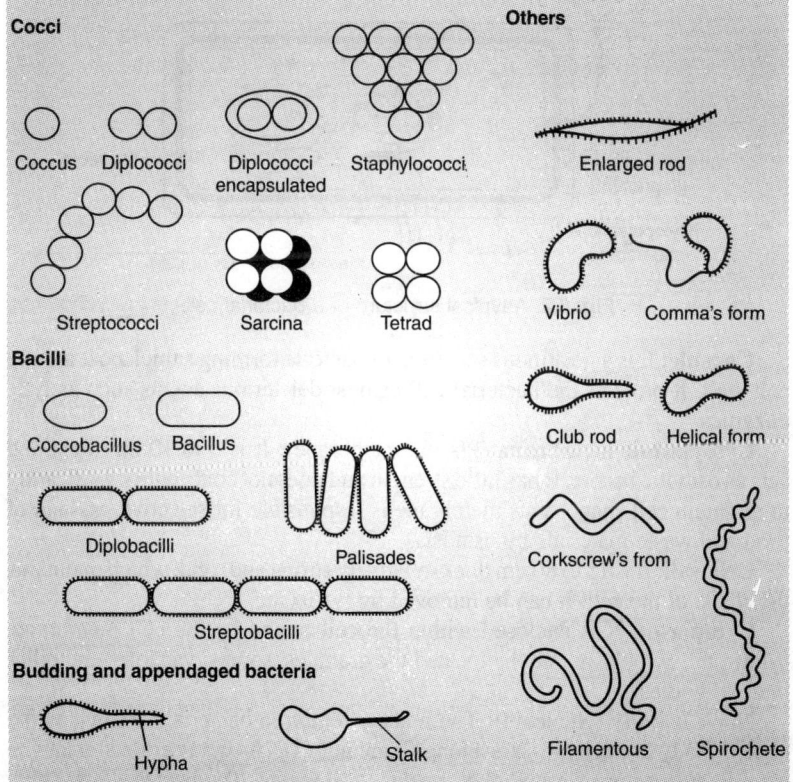

Fig. 6.1. Different shapes of bacteria.

(d) Fusiform bacilli – They are bacilli tapered at both ends.

(e) Filamentous bacilli – They are bacilli growing in long filaments.

(f) Vibrio – They are comma shaped, curved rods e.g. *Vibrio cholera.*

(g) Spirochaetes – They are thin, spiral, motile, flexible organisms with several spirals e.g. *Treponema pallidum.*

(h) Spirilla – They are longer rigid rods with several curves or coils e.g. *Spirillum minus.*

B. Bacterial Anatomy

All living organisms consist of units of protoplasm called cells. The bacterial cell consists of cytoplasm, which is enclosed within a cytoplasmic membrane and this membrane presses again at the cell wall. The structure of a bacterial cell is shown in Fig. 6.2.

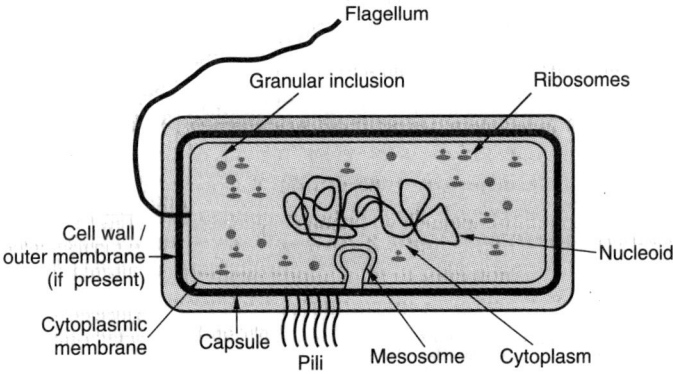

Fig. 6.2. A typical structure of a bacterial cell.

Capsule: It is a gelatinous secretion of bacteria forming a thick coat around cell wall. It protects the bacterial cell against deleterious agents such as lytic enzymes.

Cytoplasmic membrane (Plasma membrane): It is 5 to 10 nm thick and acts as osmotic barrier. It has little strength and does not contribute significantly to maintain cell shape. This membrane is responsible for selective passage of food and waste materials by osmosis.

Cell wall: It is 15 to 80 nm thick, relatively strong and rigid, which maintains the shape of the cell. It can be removed by lysozyme.

Cytoplasm: It is enclosed within the cell bound by the cell membrane. Within the cytoplasm may be located the granules, spores, vacuoles and other internal bodies.

Nuclear body (Nucleoid): The nuclear region in bacteria is known as the nuclear body or nucleoid. It is a long filament of DNA tightly coiled inside the cytoplasm but not surrounded by nuclear membrane. The bacterial cell splits into two equal parts, each with a part of the nuclear substance. This process is known as *transverse binary fission.*

Flagella: The organ of locomotion in motile bacteria is flagella. They are hair-like cytoplasmic appendages measuring 12 to 25 nm in thickness. Each flagellum originates in a spherical body located just inside the cell wall.

Fimbriae (Pili): They are short, very thin, filamentous, straight, hair-like attachments of the cell wall. They are 0.1 to 0.5 µm long and less than 4 to 8 nm thick. They are also called **pili**. They have no relation to motility. *Salmonella typhi* possesses 12 flagella and about 100 fimbriae.

Mesosomes, ribosmes and granular inclusions are the cytoplasmic contents.

Spores: Spores are highly resistant, dormant state of bacteria developed in some cells. They are resistant to heat, drying, freezing and toxic chemicals. Spores make possible survival of organisms under adverse conditions.

C. Bacterial Diseases

Some of the common bacterial diseases are shown below:

Disease	Causative bacteria
Scarlet fever	*Streptococcus pyogenes*
Pneumonia	*Streptococcus pneumoniae*
Gonorrhoea	*Neisseria gonorrhoeae*
Diphtheria	*Corynebacterium diphtheriae*
Tuberculosis	*Mycobacterium tuberculosis*
Leprosy	*Mycobactrium leprae*
Tetanus	*Clostridium tetani*
Syphilis	*Treponema pallidum*
Gastroenteritis	*Salmonella typhimurium*
Whooping cough	*Haemophilus pertussis*

FUNGI

Algae and fungi are the two subdivisions of the Phyllum Thallophyta, which consist of the most primitive plants with true roots, stems or leaves. Algae possess chlorophyll but fungi do not. Fungi are larger in size than bacteria and have more complicated structure and reproduce both sexually and asexually. Some fungi produce toxic substances called *mycotoxins*. The broad classification of fungi is given below.

A. Morphology

Two principal groups of fungi are moulds and yeasts and two sub-groups are yeast-like fungi and dimorphic fungi.

Moulds or filamentous fungi: They show tubular branched filaments called *hyphae*. The hyphae may be septate or non-septate. The hyphae intermingle to form a network called the *mycelium*. The mycelium is visible on a natural substrate or medium as colony. Moulds reproduce by formation of spores.

True yeasts: They are round or oval, unicellular fungi with filaments and reproduce by budding.

Classification of Fungi

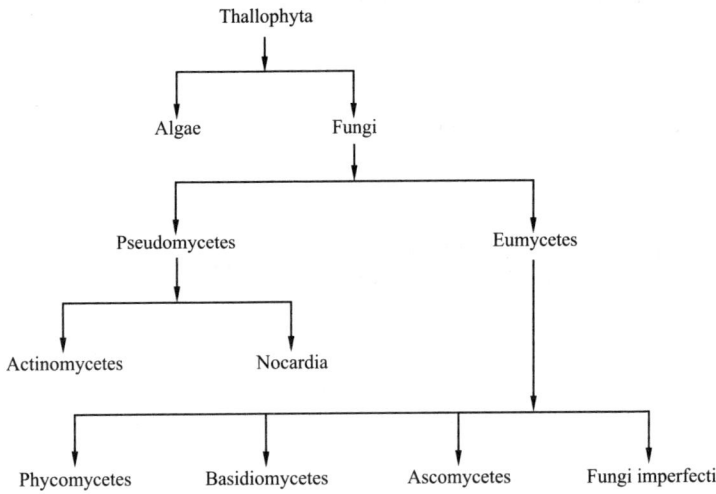

Yeast-like fungi: These fungi form pseudohypahe; they are secondary elongated buds formed from the parent bud and remain attached to it.

Dimorphic fungi: These fungi grow as moulds at room temperature (saprophytic phase) but as yeasts at 37°C or in tissues (parasitic phase).

Phycomycetes: These fungi have non-septate hyphae. They reproduce through both sexual and asexual spores.

Basidiomycetes: These are known to us as mushrooms, rusts and shelf fungi. Some are highly poisonous. These fungi show septate binucleate hyphae. Sexual spores are borne on the basidium while conidiospores are situated at the tips of phyphae. They are non-pathogenic to man.

Ascomycetes: Majority of fungi in this class have septate uninucleate hyphae. Sexual spores are ascosportes while conidiospors are borne at the tip of hyphae. Some members of this class are pathogenic to man.

Fungi imperfecti (Deuteromycetes): These fungi lack a sexual stage in their life cycle. They may be moulds, true yeasts, yeast-like or dimorphic. The two major types of asexual spores produced by these fungi are thalospores and conidiospores. Most pathogens of man belong to the class of fungi imperfecti.

B. Fungal Infections

Out of the estimated 50,000 to 200,000 species of fungi, only about 100 are known to cause infectious diseases (Mycoses) in human. Most of the pathogenic fungi live as saprophytes (organisms which obtain nutrients from dead organic matter) in the soil. Infection of human usually occurs only accidentally through contamination of cuts and abrasion by soil or by inhalation of dust containing spores or conidia.

Mycoses

These are divided into four groups differing in the level of infected tissue.

1. Systemic or deep mycoses: These primarily involve internal organs and viscera. They are often widely distributed and involve many different tissues.
2. Subcutaneous mycoses: These involve skin, subcutaneous tissue, fascia and bone.
3. Cutaneous mycoses: These involve epidermis, hair and nails. The respective fungi are called *dermatophytes* and the diseases are known as *dermatophytoses* or *dermatomycoses*.
4. Superficial mycoses: These involve only hair and the most superficial layer of epidermis. The superficial mycoses form the great bulk of mycotic diseases in India mostly due to *T. rubrum.*

Pathogenic fungi

These are:

1. Dermatophytes, which cause ring worms (superficial infection).
2. Yeast-like fungi, which are capable of invading the tissues and giving rise to generalized or systemic infections.

Most often the respiratory tract is affected as a result of inhalation of fungal spores.

Some of the more common mycoses are shown below.

Examples of Human Mycoses	
Disease	**Causative fungus**
1. Systemic Mycoses	
• Candidiasis	*Candida albicans*
• Coccidioidomycoses	*Coccidioides immitis*
• Histoplasmosis	*Histoplasma capsulatum*
• Aspergillosis	*Aspergillus fumigates*
2. Dermal Mycoses	
• Ringworm	*Microsporium audouini*
• Athlete's foot	*Epidermophyton floccosum*
• Barber's itch	*Tricophyton species*

Chemotherapy

Fungi are quite insensitive to the chemotherapeutic agents used in the treatment of bacterial infection. Effective antifungal drugs include Griseofulvin and polyene antibiotics such as Amphotericin B, Nystatin, and Flucytosin.

RICKETTSIAE

Rickettsiae are minute microorganisms having the properties between bacteria and virus. They are non-motile, non-encapsulated, don't produce spores and

capsules, and look like small bacteria readily visible with the light microscope. Like viruses they grow only in living cells. They resemble bacteria because:
1. They have cell wall.
2. They divide by binary fission.
3. They are visible with the light microscope.
4. They contain both DNA and RNA and enzymes for metabolic activities.

They differ from viruses in their large size and their inability to pass through bacteria-retaining filters.

Rickettsiae are *pleomorphic* i.e. they occur in more than one morphological form such as rod shaped, spherical, filamentous or irregularly shaped organisms. They are intestinal parasites of blood sucking arthropods such as fleas, lice, ticks, and mites. The infection is transmitted to man by the bite of these insects. They can be readily cultivated in the yolk sac of developing chick embryo. Rickettsiae are readily destroyed at 56°C and are sensitive to Tetracycline and Chloramphenicol. Penicillin and Sulfonamides are ineffective.

Rickettsial diseases of human
These are given in Table 6.2.

Table 6.2. Rickettsial diseases of human – causative organism, vector and reservoir

Disease	Causative organism	Vector	Reservoir
1. Typhus group:			
(a) Epidemic typhus	*R. prowazeki*	Louse	Man
(b) Murine typhus (endemic typhus)	*R. mooseri*	Rat flea	Rat
2. (a) Spotted fevers (Rocky mountain)	*R. rickettsi*	Tick	Tick
(b) Rickettsial pox	*R. akari*	Mites	House mice
3. Scrub fever	*R. tsusuga mushi*	Mites	Field rat, mite
4. Q fever	*Coxiella burnetii*	Infected dust	Ticks, cattle, etc.
5. Trench fever	*R. quintana*	Louse	Man

CHLAMYDIAE (Bedsonia)
Chlamydiae were considered as viruses due to their intracellular parasitism but they differ from the viruses as below:
1. They possess both DNA and RNA.
2. They contain a variety of enzymes.
3. They have ribosomes but viruses do not have ribosomes.
4. They multiply by binary fission.
5. They have muramic acid in their cell wall like bacteria.
6. They are about 200 to 300 nm in diameter and are Gram (–)ve.

Chlamydiae grow well in the yolk sac of embryonated eggs. Mice, guinea pigs and rabbits are infected by inoculation. They are rapidly killed by heat, formalin and phenol. Their multiplication is inhibited by many antibiotics. Diseases commonly caused by Chlamydiae are Psittacosis, Lymphogranuloma venereum and Trachoma.

VIRUSES

In latin 'virus' means poison. Viruses are considerably smaller than bacteria and cannot be seen with the ordinary microscope. They are nucleoprotein particles capable of multiplication in certain living cells. They differ from bacteria in (i) being intracellular obligate parasites, (ii) contain either DNA or RNA, (iii) they don't multiply by binary fission and reproduce solely through nucleic acid. Viruses vary in size from 17–400 nm. Most viruses are circular in shape but they may be round, cubical or like tadpole. Some are irregular and some are brick-shaped.

Structure

Simplest structure of viruses is nucleocapsid, which consists of a core of DNA *or* RNA encapsulated by a protein coat called a *caspid* (Fig.6.3). A higher organization shows a nucleocapsid with an envelope. The envelope contains protein. It may also contain lipid. Large viruses may consist of lipids, carbohydrates, biotin, riboflavin and copper. The DNA or RNA core may be a single or double stranded molecule. It is the essential infective substance of the virus and must be released from the protein container to initiate infection. The protein coat forms a protective covering for the nucleic acid core. It is composed of numerous morphological subunits called *capsomeres*. Each capsomere contains many protein molecules. These are the structural units. Capsomeres around the nucleic acid core may be arranged in isohedral cubic symmetry or helical symmetry. The term *virion* is applied to the complete infective virus particle.

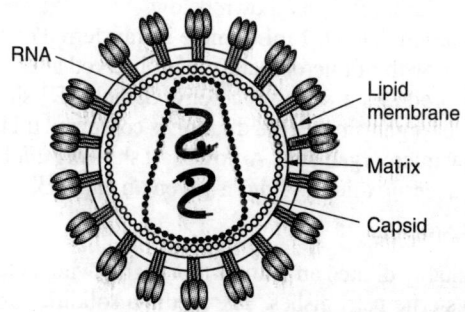

RNA — Lipid membrane — Matrix — Capsid

Fig. 6.3. Structure of a virus.

Multiplication

Bacteria multiply by binary fission while viruses enter a living cell and mix with RNA *or* DNA of the cell, break up into minute particles and are lost for some time. They reappear in the shape of minute particles that recombine and form virus particles. Viruses are cultivated in animals, yolk sac of fertile egg and tissue culture. Usually the viruses multiply in the host and they can be seen either in the nucleus or in the cytoplasm in the form of aggregate of viruses.

Resistance

Viruses are destroyed by heat. They are usually resistant to antibiotics but are inactivated by X-ray irradiation. They are more resistant to chemical disinfectants than bacteria.

ISOLATION OF MICROORGANISMS

A **pure culture** contains only one kind of microorganism but microorganisms rarely occur in pure culture. For detailed study of any bacterium it is essential that it is isolated from other microorganisms with which it might be mixed. This process is called **isolation**. Isolation and identification of disease producing organisms is the most important exercise in any bacteriological laboratory. This requires careful collection, transport and examination of clinical specimen. Specimen should be collected in sufficient quantity, in suitable containers and preserved under proper conditions. After examination the results should be interpreted by a trained bacteriologist. Proper and timely identification of pathogenic organisms helps physician to diagnose the disease and prescribe accurate and suitable therapy.

Pure Culture Techniques

1. Serial Dilution Technique

This technique is also useful in estimating number of viable microorganisms (enumeration) in water, milk, culture etc. The sample is diluted in a serial order in a sterile diluting fluid as shown below.

From each dilution A to D, 1 mL sample is transferred on to sterile culture medium and the growth of microorganisms is observed after incubating. Each single organism produces a separate colony. Sample [D] should contain the smallest number of organisms. Serial dilution is continued till the final dilution contains very few microorganisms. A flowchart showing dilution of sample in a serial order in a sterile diluting fluid is given on page 139.

2. Pour Plate Technique

The sample is suitably diluted and mixed thoroughly with melted agar medium and poured into sterile petri dishes. The medium solidifies and the plates are incubated. Colonies of bacteria develop and each colony represents a population of one and only one type of organism. Thus from a number of colonies of different bacteria (mixed culture) developed over the plate, individual colonies are picked up and further cultivated to obtain a pure culture (Fig. 6.4).

3. Streak and Spread Plate Technique

A small amount (loopful) of specimen is taken on the surface of a solid medium.

Dilution of sample in a serial order in a sterile diluting fluid

Sample (1 mL)

↓

Diluting fluid (99 mL) (1 : 100 dilution)   A

↓

(1 mL)

↓

Diluting fluid (99 mL) (1 : 10,000 dilution)   B

↓

(1 mL)

↓

Diluting fluid (9 mL) (1 : 100,000 dilution)   C

↓

(1 mL)

↓

Diluting fluid (9 mL) (1 : 1000,000 dilution) D

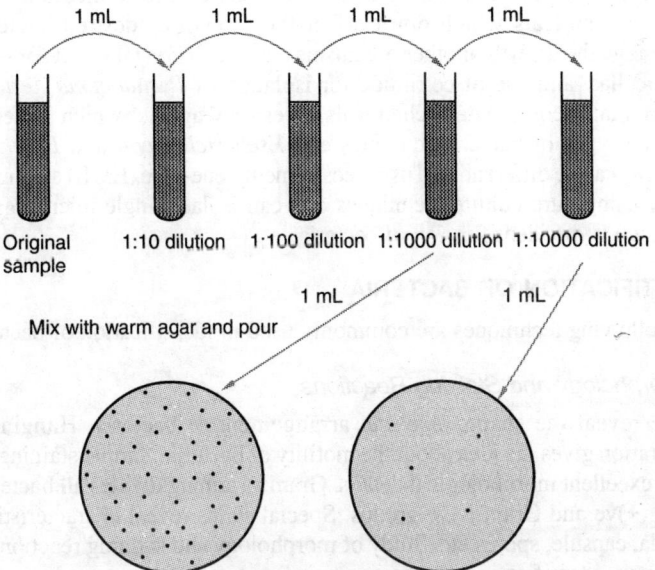

Fig. 6.4. Pour Plate Technique.

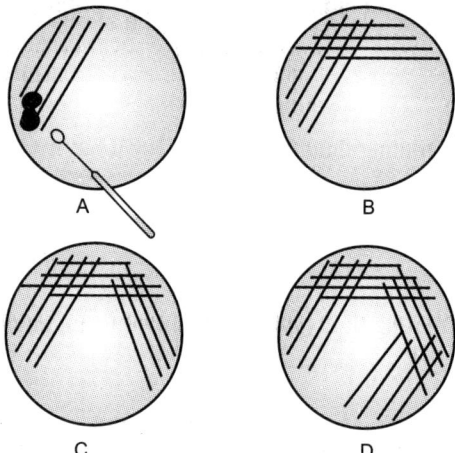

Fig. 6.5. Streak and Spread Plate Technique.

It is streaked in such a way as to provide successive dilution. Finally, well isolated colonies are obtained (Fig. 6.5).

Enrichment, selective and differential media can also be used to isolate a specific type of bacterium from a mixed population. The technique is based on the use of certain chemical agents in the media or modifying the physical conditions of incubation. Medium may be enriched with blood, serum etc to encourage growth of saprophytes or parasites. Selective medium contains specific chemicals which don't affect the growth of desired bacteria but discourage the growth of other organisms e.g. use of crystal violet for isolation of brucellas, and use of cetrimide for isolation of *Pseudomona aeruginosa*. Differential media contain chemicals, dyes or reagents, which differentiate between types of bacterial colonies e.g. *Escherichia coli* and *Enterobacter aerogens* can be differentiated using eosin-methylene-blue (EMB) agar medium.

By using pure culture techniques one can isolate single microorganisms. Next step is the identification of bacteria.

IDENTIFICATION OF BACTERIA

The following techniques are commonly used in identification of bacteria.

A. Morphology and Staining Reactions

These reveal the shape, size and arrangement of bacteria. Hanging drop preparation gives the idea about the motility of bacteria. Simple staining brings about excellent morphological details. Gram's staining divides all bacteria into Gram (+)ve and Gram (-)ve groups. Special stains reveal characteristics like flagella, capsule, spores etc. Study of morphology and staining reactions helps in primary identification of microorganisms.

B. Cultural Characteristics

Under appropriate cultural conditions bacteria show characteristic type of growth. Colonies or growth formed on different solid media gives important information about the unknown microorganisms. Colonies are observed in respect of size, margin, elevation, type of growth and type of liquefaction (Fig. 6.6).

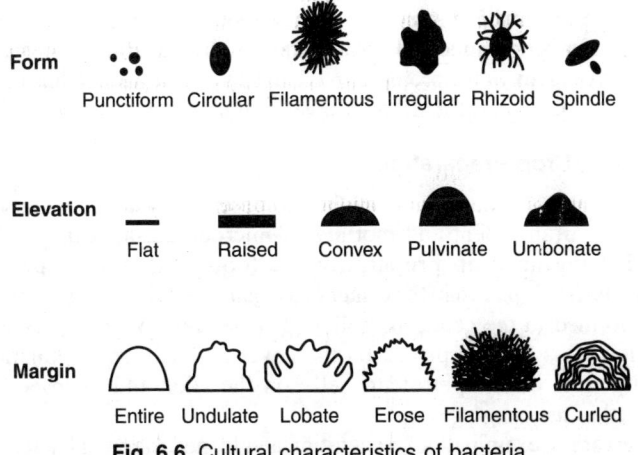

Fig. 6.6. Cultural characteristics of bacteria.

C. Resistance

Resistance of microorganisms to heat, disinfectants, antibiotics etc helps in their differentiation and identification. *Streptococcus faecalis* can tolerate heat at 60°C for 30 minutes and *Clostridium* spores can withstand boiling for varying periods.

D. Metabolism

Bacteria can be classified and differentiated on the basis of requirements of oxygen, carbon dioxide, capacity to form pigments and power of hemolysis.

E. Biochemical Reactions

The organisms having same morphology and cultural characteristics may have marked differences in their biochemical reactions. Common biochemical tests include sugar fermentation, indole fermentation, methyl red test, Voges-Proskauer test, citrate utilization, nitrate reduction, urease test, hydrogen sulfide production, catalase production, oxidase reaction and growth in KCN. These biochemical tests provide further clues to the identity of the microorganisms.

F. Other Tests

These include serological reactions like antigenic characteristics, fluorescent microscopy, phage and bacteriocin typing, animal pathogenicity and toxigenicity.

Modern methods for rapid identification of microorganisms include counter-current immuno-electrophoresis, gas liquid chromatography (GLC), high pressure liquid chromatography (HPLC), microcalorimetry, luminescence biometry, radiorespirometry etc.

STAINING TECHNIQUES OF MICROORGANISMS OF COMMON DISEASES

Bacteria are too small in size to be seen without the use of microscope. The problem is further complicated because most of the bacteria are colourless and the refractive index of the protoplasm is same as that of water. Thus bacteria in their natural state are difficult to observe even under microscope.

A. Hanging Drop Preparation

This is a simple and convenient method to observe *live* microorganisms. The size, shape arrangement and motility of microorganisms can be observed through hanging drop preparation. A loopful of the suspension of microorganisms is placed in the center of a clean cover slip. A ring of petroleum jelly is formed in the center of hollow ground slide. With depression slide down, the glass slide is placed on the cover slip and gently inverted. The coverslip rests on the petroleum jelly on the slide and microbes remain suspended in the *hanging* drop.

Observation, examination, recognition and identification of bacteria can be possible if the organisms are stained so that they stand out as coloured objects in contrast with the background, which is nearly colourless. For staining of microorganisms many organic dyes are used. These dyes are acidic, basic or neutral. Commonly used dyes include eosin or sodium eosinate (acidic), methylene blue (basic), crystal violet, safranin etc.

Staining is either simple or differential. In simple staining all cells take up the same colour of a single dye such as fuchsin or methylene blue. In differential staining e.g. Gram's stain, the cells are differentiated by two contrasting colours (red & blue or pink & violet). Certain special stains are used for staining of particular components or bacterial cells or specific organ e.g. capsular stain, flagellar stain etc.

Smear Preparation and Simple Staining

When bacterial detail is to be observed, more specific stains are necessary and this can be achieved by smear preparation and simple staining. A bacterial *smear* is a dried preparation of bacterial cells on a glass slide. In a bacterial smear that has been properly processed (i) the bacteria are evenly spread out on the slide in such a concentration that they are adequately separated from one another, (ii) the bacteria are not washed off the slide during staining, and (iii) bacterial form is not distorted.

In making a smear, bacteria from either a broth culture or an agar slant or plate may be used. If a slant or plate is used, a small amount of bacterial growth is transferred to a drop of water on a glass slide (Fig. 6.7) and mixed. The

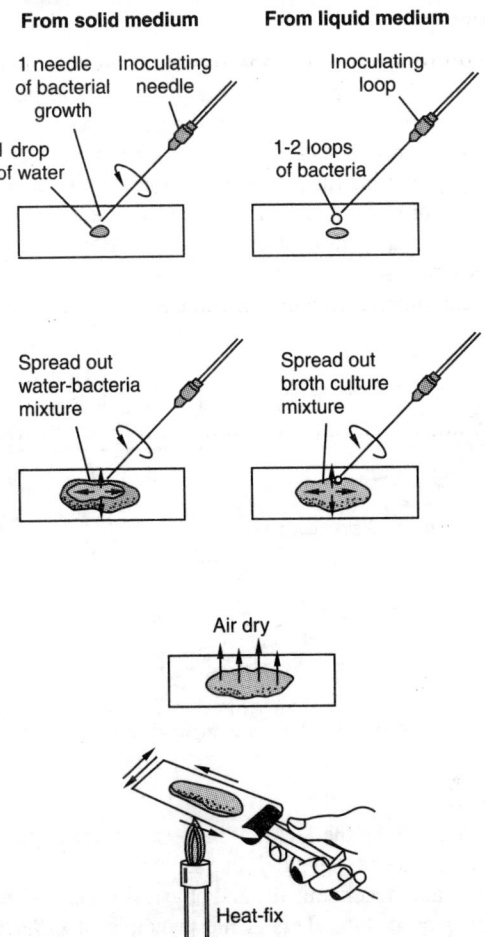

Fig. 6.7. Steps involved in smear preparation.

mixture is then spread out evenly over a large area on the slide. One of the most common errors in smear preparation from agar cultures is the use of too large an inoculum. This invariably results in the occurrence of large aggregates of bacteria piled on top of one another.

If the medium is liquid, place one or two loops of the medium directly on the slide and spread the bacteria over a large area. Allow the slide to air dry at room temperature. After the smear is dry, the next step is to attach the bacteria to the slide by heat-fixing. This is accomplished by gentle heating, passing the slide several times through the hot portion of the flame of a Bunsen burner. Most bacteria can be fixed to the slide and killed in this way without serious distortion of cell structure.

B. Simple Staining

The use of a single stain or dye to create contrast between the bacteria and the background is referred to as **simple staining**. Its chief value lies in its simplicity and ease of use. Simple staining is often employed when information about cell shape, size, and arrangement is desired. In this procedure, one places the heat-fixed slide on a staining rack, covers the smear with a small amount of the desired stain for the proper amount of time, washes the stain off with water for a few seconds, and, finally, blots it dry (Fig. 6.8). Basic dyes such as crystal violet (20 to 30 seconds staining time), carbol fuchsin (5 to 10 seconds staining time), or methylene blue (1 minute staining time) are often used.

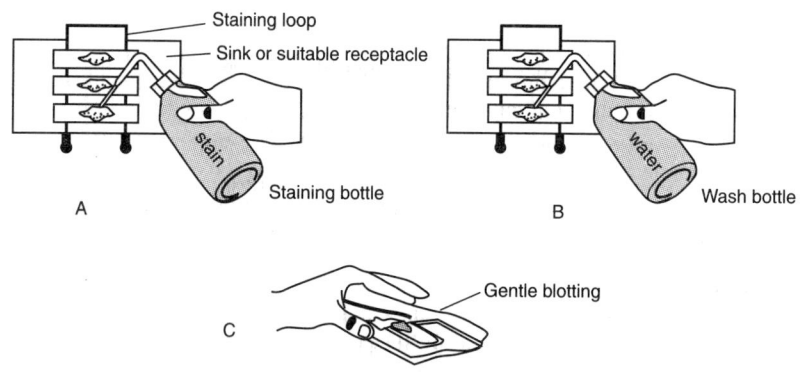

Fig. 6.8. Steps in simple staining.

C. Gram Staining

Simple staining depends on the fact that bacteria differ chemically from their surroundings and thus can be stained in contrast with their environment. Bacteria also differ from one another chemically and physically and may react differently to a given staining procedure. This is the principle of *differential staining*. Differential staining can distinguish between types of bacteria.

The Gram stain (named after Christian Gram, Danish scientist and physician, 1853–1938) is the most useful and widely employed differential stain in bacteriology. It divides bacteria into two groups- Gram negative and Gram positive.

(a) Traditional Gram-Staining Technique

This technique involves staining with the basic dye, crystal violet. This is the primary stain. It is followed by treatment with an iodine solution, which functions as a mordant; that is, it increases the interaction between the bacterial cell and the dye so that the dye is more tightly bound or the cell is more strongly stained. The smear is then decolourized by washing with 95% ethanol or isopropanol-acetone. Gram-positive bacteria retain the crystal violet-iodine complex when washed with the decolourizer, whereas Gram-negative bacteria lose their crystal violet-iodine complex and become colourless. Finally, the smear is counter-stained with a basic dye, different in colour than crystal violet. This counter- stain is usually safranin. The safranin will stain the colourless, Gram-negative bacteria pink but does not alter the dark purple colour of the Gram-positive bacteria. The end result is that Gram-positive bacteria are deep purple in colour in contrast while Gram-negative bacteria are pinkish to red in colour (Fig. 6.9).

Steps in traditional Gram staining

1. Prepare heat-fixed smears of microbe e.g. *E. coli, S. aureus,* and the mixture of both.
2. Place the slides on the staining rack and flood the smears with crystal violet and allow to stand for 30 seconds.
3. Rinse with water for 5 seconds then cover with Gram's iodine mordant and allow to stand for 1 minute.
4. Rinse with water for 5 seconds.
5. Decolourize with 95% ethanol for 15 to 30 seconds. Do not decolourize too long. Add the decolourizer drop by drop until the crystal violet fails to wash from the slide. Alternatively, the smears may be decolourized for 30 to 60 seconds with a mixture of isopropanol-acetone (3:1 *v/v*).
6. Rinse with water for 5 seconds then counterstain with safranin for about 60 to 80 seconds.
7. Rinse with water for 5 seconds.
8. Blot dry with filter paper and examine under oil immersion.
9. Gram-positive organisms stain blue to purple; Gram-negative organisms stain pink to red.

(b) Three step Gram staining

Recently Difco Laboratories has introduced reagents for a three-step Gram stain. The advantages include less reagent usage versus conventional stains, reduced chance of over decolourization, and saved time. The recommended procedure is as follows:

1. Flood the smear with Gram crystal violet primary stain and stain for 1 minute.
2. Wash off the crystal violet with cold water then flood the slide with Gram's iodine mordant and allow standing for 1 minute.
3. Wash off the mordant with safranin decolourizer/counterstain solution. Then add more decolourizer/counterstain solution to the slide and stain for 20 to 50 seconds.
4. Wash off the decolourizer/counterstain with cold water then either blot or air dry.

Some important differences between Gram positive and Gram negative bacteria are shown in Table 6.3.

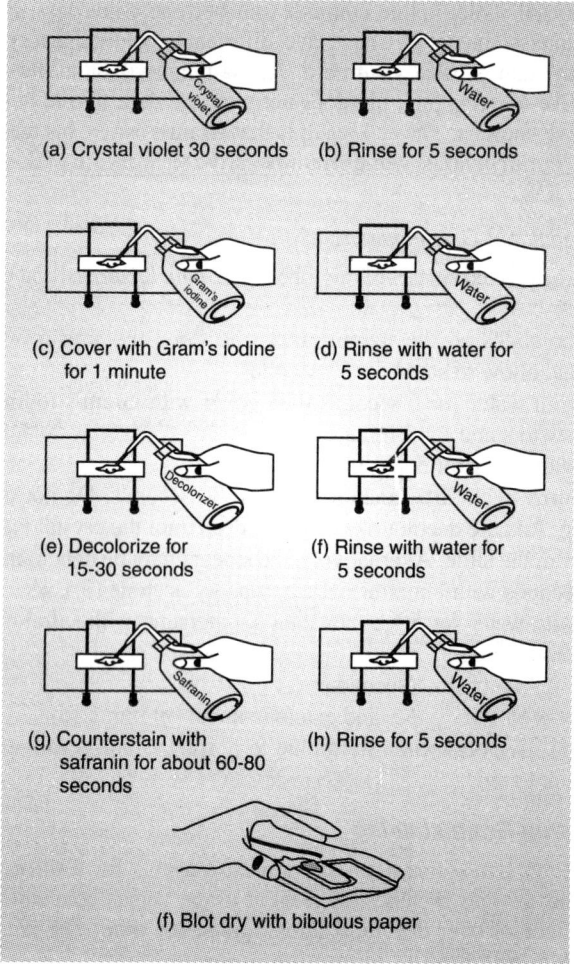

(a) Crystal violet 30 seconds   (b) Rinse for 5 seconds

(c) Cover with Gram's iodine for 1 minute   (d) Rinse with water for 5 seconds

(e) Decolorize for 15-30 seconds   (f) Rinse with water for 5 seconds

(g) Counterstain with safranin for about 60-80 seconds   (h) Rinse for 5 seconds

(f) Blot dry with bibulous paper

Fig. 6.9. Different steps involved in Gram staining.

In general, Gram negative organisms are more pathogenic and harmful. Examples of some Gram positive and Gram negative organisms are give below:

Gram positive organisms	Gram negative organisms
Streptococcus pneumoniae	*Corynebacterium diphtheriae*
Staphylococcus aureus	*Neisseria gonorrhoeae*
Bacillus anthracis	*Escherichia coli*
Streptococcus hemolyticus	*Vibrio cholerae*
Clostridium tetani	*Haemophilus influenzae*

Table 6.3. Differences between Gram positive and Gram negative bacteria

Property	Gram positive	Gram negative
Ratio of RNA to DNA in cell	8 : 1	Almost equal
Susceptibility to sulfonamide, drugs and penicillin	Marked	Much less
Susceptibility to anionic detergents, basic dyes, lysozyme, iodine	Marked	Much less
Digestion by trypsin or pepsin	Resistant	Susceptible
Susceptibility by lysis by complement	Slight	Marked
Susceptibility to action of proteolytic enzymes and alkalies	Resistant	Susceptible
Lipids in cell wall	Little (3%)	Much (20%)
Nutritional requirements	More complex	Simple
Mesosomes	Present	Rare or absent
Aromatic and S-containing amino acids in cell wall	None	Numerous

Medical Application

Gram staining is the single most useful test in the clinical microbiology laboratory. It is the differential staining procedure most commonly used for the direct examination of specimens and bacterial colonies because it has a broad staining spectrum. The Gram stain is the first differential test run on a bacterial specimen brought into the laboratory for specific identification. The staining spectrum includes almost all bacteria, many fungi, and parasites such as *Trichomonas*, *Strongyloides*, and miscellaneous protozoan cysts. The significant exceptions include *Treponema*, *Mycoplasma*, *Chlamydia*, and *Rickettsia*, which are too small to be seen by light microscopy or lack a cell wall.

D. Acid-Fast Staining (Ziehl-Neelsen and Kinyoun)

A few species of bacteria in the genera Mycobacterium and Nocardia, and the parasite Cryptosporidium do not readily stain with simple stains. However, these microorganisms can be stained by heating them with carbol fuchsin. The heat drives the stain into the cells. Once the microorganisms have taken up the carbol fuchsin, they are not easily decolourized by acid-alcohol, and hence are termed acid-fast. This acid-fastness is due to the high lipid content (mycolic acid) in the cell wall of these microorganisms.

The Ziehl-Neelsen acid-fast staining procedure (developed by Franz Ziehl, a German bacteriologist, and Friedrich Neelsen, a German pathologist, in the late 1800s) is a very useful differential staining technique that makes use of this difference in retention of carbol fuchsin. Acid-fast microorganisms will retain this dye and appear red. Microorganisms that are not acid-fast, termed non-acid-fast, will appear blue or brown due to the counterstaining with methylene blue after they have been decolourized by the acid-alcohol (Fig. 6.10).

(a) Ziehl-Neelsen (Hot Stain) method

This method of staining includes following steps:

1. Prepare a smear of given microorganism then allow the smear to air dry and then heat-fix.
2. Place the slide on a hot plate (within a chemical hood), and cover the smear with a piece of paper toweling that has been cut to the same size as the microscope slide. Saturate the paper with Ziehl's carbol fuchsin.
3. Heat for 3 to 5 minutes. Do not allow the slide to dry out, and avoid excess flooding. Also, prevent boiling by adjusting the hot plate to a proper temperature.
4. Remove the slide, allow it to cool, and rinse with water for 30 seconds.
5. Decolourize by adding acid-alcohol drop by drop until the slide remains only slightly pink.
6. Rinse with water for 5 seconds then counter-stain with alkaline methylene blue for about 2 minutes.
7. Then rinse with water for 30 seconds and blot dry with filter paper.

Acid-fast organisms stain red; the background and other organisms stain blue or brown.

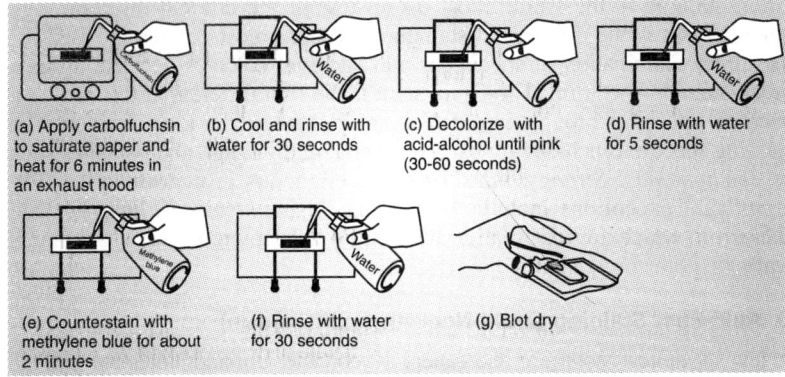

(a) Apply carbolfuchsin to saturate paper and heat for 6 minutes in an exhaust hood

(b) Cool and rinse with water for 30 seconds

(c) Decolorize with acid-alcohol until pink (30-60 seconds)

(d) Rinse with water for 5 seconds

(e) Counterstain with methylene blue for about 2 minutes

(f) Rinse with water for 30 seconds

(g) Blot dry

Fig. 6.10. Steps involved in Acid-fast staining.

(b) Kinyoun (Cold Stain) method

This may be used instead of/or in addition to the Ziehl-Neelsen procedure.

1. Heat-fix the slide as mentioned previously then flood the slide for 5 minutes with carbol fuchsin prepared with Tergitol No. 7 (heat is not necessary).
2. Decolourize with acid-alcohol and wash with tap water. Repeat this step until no more colour runs off the slide.
3. Counterstain with alkaline methylene blue for 2 minutes. Wash and blot dry.

Acid-fast organisms stain red; the background and other organisms stain blue.

D. Negative Staining

Negative staining is satisfactory when simple observations on bacterial morphology and size are made. It is called *negative* staining because in this method bacteria are not stained hence they appear as bright objects in contrast with the stained (coloured) background. Negative staining is particularly suitable for capsules, which appear as clean halo between refractile outline of cell wall and greyish background of Indian ink.

Sometimes it is convenient to determine overall bacterial morphology without the use of harsh staining or heat-fixing techniques that change the shape of cells. This might be the case when the bacterium does not stain well (for example, some of the spirochetes) or when it is desirable to confirm observations made on the shape and size of bacteria observed in either a wet-mount or hanging drop slide. Negative staining is also good for viewing capsules.

Negative, indirect, or *background staining* is achieved by mixing bacteria with an acidic stain such as nigrosin, India ink, or eosin, and then spreading out the mixture on a slide to form a film. The above stains will not penetrate and stain the bacterial cells due to repulsion between the negative charge of the stains and the negatively charged bacterial wall. Instead, these stains either produce a deposit around the bacteria or produce a dark background so that the bacteria appear as unstained cells with a clear area around them (Fig. 6.11).

The procedure for negative staining includes following steps:

1. Using an inoculating loop, apply a small amount of bacteria to one end of a clean microscope slide.
2. Add 1 to 2 loops of nigrosin, India ink or eosin solution to the bacteria and mix thoroughly.
3. Spread the mixture over the slide using a second slide. The second slide should be held at a 45° angle so that the bacteria-nigrosin solution spreads across its edge. The slide is then pushed across the surface of the first slide in order to form a smear that is thick at one end and thin at the other.
4. Allow the smear to air dry. Do not heat-fix.
5. Use the oil immersion lens to observe bacterial species.

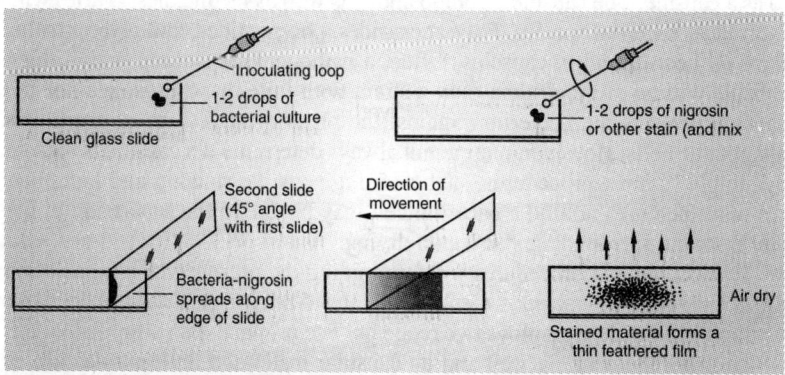

Fig. 6.11. Steps involved in Negative staining.

Medical Application

Treponema pallidum is the spirochete that causes the sexually transmitted disease *syphilis*. This bacterium is a very delicate cell that is easily distorted by heat-fixing; thus, negative staining is the procedure of choice in the clinical laboratory.

E. Endospore Staining (Schaeffer-Fulton Or Wirtz-Conklin)

Bacteria in genera such as *Bacillus* and *Clostridium* produce quite a resistant structure capable of surviving for long periods in an unfavorable environment and then giving rise to a new bacterial cell. This structure is called an *endospore* since it develops within the bacterial cell. Endospores are spherical to elliptical in shape and may be either smaller or larger than the parent bacterial cell. Endospore position within the cell is characteristic and may be central, subterminal, or terminal.

Endospores do not stain easily, but once stained, they strongly resist decolourization. This property is the basis of the Schaeffer-Fulton or Wirtz-Conklin method of staining endospores. The endospores are stained with malachite green. Heat is used to provide stain penetration. The rest of the cell is then decolourized and counter-stained a light red with safranin. The spores, both endospores and free spores, stain green; vegetative cells stain red.

Medical Application

Only a few bacteria produce endospores. Those of medical importance include *Bacillus anthracis* (anthrax), *Clostridium tetani* (tetanus), *C. botulinium* (botulism), and *C. perfringens* (gas gangrene). In the clinical laboratory, the location and size of endospores vary with the species; thus, they are often of value in identifying bacteria.

F. Capsule Staining

Many bacteria have a slimy layer surrounding them, which is usually referred to as a capsule. The capsule's composition, as well as its thickness, varies with individual bacterial species. Polysaccharides, polypeptides, and glycoproteins have all been found in capsules. Often, a pathogenic bacterium with a thick capsule will be more virulent than a strain with little or no capsule since the capsule protects the bacterium against the phagocytic activity of the host's phagocytic cells. However, one cannot always determine if a capsule is present by simple staining procedures, such as using negative staining and India ink. An unstained area around a bacterial cell may be due to the separation of the cell from the surrounding stain upon drying.

Two convenient procedures for determining the presence of a capsule are *Anthony's capsule staining method* and the *Graham & Evans procedure*. Anthony's procedure employs two reagents. The primary stain is crystal violet, which gives the bacterial cell and its capsular material a dark purple colour. Unlike the cell, the capsule is non-ionic and the primary stain cannot adhere.

Copper sulfate is the decolourizing agent. It removes excess primary stain as well as colour from the capsule. At the same time, the copper sulfate acts as a counter-stain by being absorbed into the capsule and turning it a light blue or pink. In this procedure, smears should not be heat-fixed since shrinkage is likely to occur and create a clear zone around the bacterium, which can be mistaken for a capsule.

Steps in Graham & Evans method

1. Thoroughly clean the slide to be used with alcohol.
2. Mix two loopfuls of culture with 1 to 2 drops of India ink at one end of the slide.
3. Spread out the drop using a second slide in the same way one prepares a thin smear.
4. Dry the smear and gently rinse with distilled water.
5. Stain for 1 minute with Gram's crystal violet then rinse again with water.
6. Stain for 1.5 minutes with safranin stain, rinse with water and blot dry.
7. If a capsule is present then pink to red bacteria are surrounded by a clear zone. The background is blue-black.

Medical Application

Many bacteria e.g., *Bacillus anthracis* (anthrax), *Streptococcus mutans* (tooth decay), *Streptococcus pneumoniae* (pneumonia) and the fungus *Cryptococcus neoformans* (cryptococcosis) contain a gelatinous covering called a capsule. In the clinical laboratory, demonstrating the presence of a capsule is a means of diagnosis and determining the organism's virulence, the degree to which a pathogen can cause disease.

G. Flagella Staining

Bacterial flagella are fine, thread-like organelles of locomotion. They are slender (about 10 to 30 nm in diameter) and can be seen directly using only the electron microscope. In order to observe them with the light microscope, the thickness of the flagella are increased by coating them with mordant such as tannic acid and potassium alum, and staining them with basic fuchsin (Gray method), para rosaniline (Leifson method), silver nitrate (West method), or crystal violet (Difco's method). Although flagella staining procedures are difficult to carry out, they often provide information about the presence and location of flagella, which is of great value in bacterial identification. *Difco's Spot Test Flagella stain* employs an alcoholic solution of crystal violet as the primary stain, and tannic acid and aluminum potassium sulfate as mordants. As the alcohol evaporates during the staining procedure, the crystal violet forms a precipitate around the flagella, thereby increasing their apparent size.

Medical Application

In the clinical laboratory, the presence, number and arrangement of flagella are useful in identifying bacterial species. Important pathogens that are motile due to the presence of flagella include *Bordetella pertussis* (whooping cough), *Listeria monocytogenes* (meningoencephalitis), *Proteus vulgaris* (urinary tract infections, bacteremia, pneumonia), *Pseudomonas aeruginosa* (skin and wound infections), *Salmonella typhi* (typhus or typhoid fever), and *Vibrio cholerae* (cholera).

Transmission of communicable diseases, their prevention and cure, immunization; and microbial technology are based on the principles of microbiology. Fundamental knowledge of microbiology is essential for a community pharmacist in understanding various infectious diseases, their control and treatment; as well as hygiene and public health.

Communicable Diseases

INTRODUCTION

Disease is an illness, defined as a state of disorder in which the normal functioning of the body is disturbed. Diseases, which are transmitted directly or indirectly from one person to another are called *communicable diseases*. Communicable diseases are also known as *contagious* or *transmissible diseases*. These diseases result from infection of pathogens including some viruses, bacteria, fungi, protozoa, multi-cellular parasites and even from contagion of peculiar proteins i.e. prions. Practicing hygiene and improving the living standard of the general public can prevent these diseases. A pharmacist, being in direct contact with the general public, is in a better position to educate the people about the general aspects of communicable diseases, their causes, modes of spread of these diseases, their prevention and control.

CLASSIFICATION OF INFECTIOUS DISEASES

On the basis of organisms causing infection, communicable diseases have been classified as shown in Table 7.1. Some of the communicable diseases of importance in India are summarized in Table 7.2.

RESPIRATORY TRACT INFECTIONS

(a) Chickenpox (Varicella)

It is a mild and acute, communicable viral infection occurring mostly in children under 10 years age. It is characterized by vesicular skin rash, which may be accompanied by fever and malaise. It occurs worldwide sporadically, endemically or epidemically.

Table 7.1. Classification of communicable diseases on the basis of organisms causing infection

Viral diseases	Bacterial diseases	Nematodes diseases	Protozoan parasites diseases
• Chicken pox	• Cholera	• Hook worm	• Malarial
• Measles	• Diphtheria	infestation	
• Influenza	• Leprosy	• Filariasis	
• Poliomyelitis	• Syphilis		
• Hepatitis	• Gonorrhea		
• Rabies	• Whooping cough		
• AIDS	(Pertussis)		
	• Tuberculosis		
	• Typhoid		
	• Tetanus		
	• Trachoma		
	• Food poisoning		
	• Plague		

Causative organism

Filterable virus, *Varicella zoster* (V-Z).

Incubation period

14 to 16 days.

Mode of transmission

Source of infection is the infected persons. Chicken pox is an airborne disease transmitted easily through droplet infection, mostly by face-to-face (personal) contact or through direct contact with secretions from the rash. The virus can cross the placental barrier and infect the fetus (congenital varicella). Infected articles also spread the infection. Patient infected with chicken pox is infectious one to two days before the rash appears and contagious period continues for four to five days after the appearance of the rash or until all lesions have crusted over. Crusted lesions are not contagious.

Prevention and control

Prevention: The only preventive measure is to avoid contact with a patient of chickenpox. The usual control measures are notification, isolation of cases for about 6 days and disinfection of articles soiled by nasal and throat discharges. The disease confers lifelong immunity. The varicella virus is susceptible to disinfectants such as chlorine bleach, desiccation, heat and detergents; hence these viruses are relatively easy to kill. Maintenance of good hygiene is necessary and daily cleaning of skin with warm water avoids secondary bacterial infection.

Vaccine: Initially there was no vaccine for chicken pox. But in 1974 Michiaki Takahashi developed a varicella vaccine from Oka strain and it was

Table 7.2. Summary of communicable diseases

Disease	Causative organisms	Symptoms	Incubation period	Mode of transmission	Prevention	Treatment
1. Chicken Pox	*Varicella zoster*	Vesicular skin rash with malaise and fever	14 to 16 days	Droplet infection	Isolation and quarantine of infected person; Varicella vaccine	Antiviral drugs
2. Measles	Paramyxovirus	Three Cs – Cough, Coryza, Conjunctivitis accompanied by fever	9 to 12 days	Droplet infection	Isolation and quarantine of infected person; Measles vaccine alone as well as in combination with mumps and rubella	No specific treatment is available
3. Influenza	Myxoviruses	Fever, headache, chills, sore throat, cough, weakness and severe aches	18 to 72 hours	Droplet infection	Isolation and quarantine of infected person; prophylactic immunization with Influenza vaccine	Antiviral drugs, particularly neuraminidase inhibitors (Tamiflu and Relenza)
4. Diphtheria	*Corynebacterium diphtheria*	Inflammation of nose, throat and tonsils	2 to 5 days	Droplet infection	Artificial active immunization with alum precipitated diphtheria toxoid	Anti-diphtheria serum and antibiotics such as penicillin
5. Whooping cough	*Bordetella pertussis* or *Haemophillus pertussis*	Fever, cold and irritating cough	7 to 14 days	Droplet infection and direct contact	Isolation, treatment and disinfection of discharges	Active immunization with DPT vaccine

(Contd.)

Disease	Causative organisms	Symptoms	Incubation period	Mode of transmission	Prevention	Treatment
6. Tuberculosis	*Mycobacterium tuberculosis*	Cough, chronic fever, chest pain, weakness and loss of weight; blood in sputum in later stage	4 to 6 weeks for primary lesions, disease develops in a period of up to 1 year	Through droplets and vomits	Sanitation and health education; active immunization with BCG vaccine	Anti-tubercular drugs such as Isoniazid, Rifampicin, Ethambutol, Pyrazinamide and Streptomycin
7. Poliomyelitis	*Poliovirus*	Paralysis of voluntary muscles of lower extremities	7 to 14 days	Faeco-oral route	Active immunization of children with polio vaccine	Bed rest and affected limb should be supported
8. Hepatitis	*Hepatitis A virus*	Fever and dark yellow urine, yellowish tinge in eyes and general paleness	2 to 5 weeks	Food and water	Improved sanitation; active immunization with Hepatitis (rDNA) vaccine	No specific treatment; patient is suggested to take rest and avoid fatty food and alcohol
9. Cholera	*Vibrio cholerae*	Severe watery diarrhea, vomiting, leg cramps, thirst	1 to 5 days	Food and water	Disinfection and proper sanitation	Management of dehydration by plenty of fluids and oral rehydration solution
10. Typhoid	*Salmonella typhi*	Severe headache, fever with low pulse, dry white coated tongue	14 to 21 days	Food and water	Isolation and treatment of patient; TAB vaccine	Widal test for diagnosis, treat with appropriate antibiotics such as fluoroquinolones and cephalosporins

(Contd.)

Disease	Causative organisms	Symptoms	Incubation period	Mode of transmission	Prevention	Treatment
11. Food poisoning	Exotoxin of *Clostridium botulinum*	Dyspepsia, blurring of vision, muscle weakness without fever	12 to 36 hours	Food	Active immunization with botulism toxoid	Antibiotics; Guanidine hydrochloride
12. Hookworm infestation	*Ancylostoma duodenale* and *Necator americanus*	Severe anemia, joint pains, dyspepsia, oedema and eosinophelia	6 weeks	Direct contact	Health education and hygiene	Benzimidazole (Albendazole, Mebendazole); Alcopar (bephenium hydroxy naphthoate); tetra-chloroethylene
13. Plague	*Pasturella pestis*	High fever, inflammation of lymphatic glands, formation of buboes	3 to 6 days (Bubonic plague); 1–4 days (Pneumonic plague)	Rat flea act as vector	Isolation of patients; anti-rat campaign Mass vaccination with killed plague vaccine	Antibiotic (Streptomycin, Gentamycin, Doxycycline, Ciprofloxacin)
14. Malaria	*Plasmodium vivax*, *P. falciparum*, *P. malariae* and *P. ovale*	Cold stage, hot stage, sweating stage	10 to 30 days	Bite of infected anopheles mosquitoes	Anti-mosquito measures and protection from mosquito bites	Anti-malarial drugs (Chloroquine, Quinine, Mefloquine, Halofantrine, etc.)

(Contd.)

Disease	Causative organisms	Symptoms	Incubation period	Mode of transmission	Prevention	Treatment
15. Filariasis	*Wucherria bancrofti* and *W. malayi*	Elephantitis	—	Culex fatigans and Mansonides mosquitoes bite	Anti-mosquito measures and protection from mosquito bites	Diethylcarbamazine
16. Rabies	Neurotropic RNA virus of *Rhabdovirus* group	Hydrophobia (almost always fatal)	10 days to 8 months	Bite of a rabid animal (Zoonotic disease)	Proper washing of wound with disinfectant; anti-rabies hyperimmune serum	Anti-rabies vaccine
17. Trachoma	*Chlamydiae trachomatis*	Inflammation of conjunctiva and cornea	5 to 12 days	Eye to eye (direct or indirect)	Health education	Sulphacetamide eye drops and Tetracycline eye ointments
18. Tetanus	Endotoxin of *Clostridium tetani*	Painful spasms and twitching of the jaw muscles	3 to 21 days	Through injury and invasion	Cleaning of wounds with 3% iodine solution; active immunization with triple vaccine (diphtheria, pertussis and tetanus)	Anti Tetanus Serum (ATS) or Human Tetanus Immunoglobulin; Penicillin and Tetracycline
19. Leprosy	*Mycobacterium leprae*	Characteristic lesions on skin, muscle weakness and paralysis	6 months to 8 years	Droplet infection	Early diagnosis; notification and isolation of patient	Chemotherapy (Rifampicin, Dapsone, Clofazimine)

(Contd.)

Disease	Causative organisms	Symptoms	Incubation period	Mode of transmission	Prevention	Treatment
20. Syphilis	*Trepenoma pallidum*	Enlarged heart and blood vessels, blindness, deafness, insanity and sterility	9 to 90 days	Sexual intercourse, blood transfusion and through placenta	Health education	Long-acting penicillins
21. Gonorrhea	*Neisseria gonorrhoeae*	Inflamed urethra, painful micturition and purulent discharge	2 days to 2 weeks	Sexual intercourse	Health education	Penicillin antibiotics in combination with Probenecid
22. AIDS	*Human immunodeficiency virus*	Destruction of immune system	6 months to 10 years	Sexual intercourse, blood transfusion and through placenta	Health education	Anti-retroviral drugs

available in U.S. since 1995. According to I.P. 2007, Varicella Vaccine is a freeze-dried preparation of a suitable attenuated strain of *Herpesvirus varicellae*. Varicella vaccine does not provide life-long protection and a second dose is needed after five years of initial immunization.

Treatment

The disease is self-limited and hence no treatment is required. The immune system clears the virus from the body. The patient suffering from serious complications needs hospitalization. Usually the treatment is symptomatic and Calamine Lotion is applied topically because it is a topical barrier preparation.

The disease confers life-long immunity.

(b) Measles (Rubeola)

Measles is a highly infectious viral disease of childhood. It is considered as a 'pediatric priority' in the developing countries. It is characterized by fever; catarrhal symptoms of the upper respiratory tract and red eye; known as three **Cs** – cough, coryza (runny nose) and conjunctivitis followed by a generalized maculopapular erythematous rashes. It is also known as *rubeola* or *morbilli*. Rubeola should not be confused with Rubella (German Measles), which is not related to measles.

Causative organism

Measles is caused by an RNA paramyxo virus particularly belonging to the genus *Morbillivirus*. Paramyxoviruses are typically consisting of a single stranded, negative sense RNA, which is enveloped in viral protein. The virus belongs to myxo-virus group present in nasopharyngeal secretions and in blood of infected individuals.

Incubation period

9–12 days.

Mode of transmission

Transmission occurs from person to person mainly by droplet infection, droplet nuclei and direct contact. The case of measles is infectious from 4 days before and 5 days after the appearance of rash. Occasionally, recently contaminated articles may transmit the infection. The rash is bright pink or red in color. It appears on the 3rd to 4th day after the onset of fever, first noticed behind the ear and on the face. It then descends downwards and covers the whole body within two days. The rash fades away within a week leaving a brownish coloration.

Measles and chickenpox may occur together. First infection diminishes the severity of the rash due to second infection.

Care

Most patients of measles recover without specific treatment. Drugs are required only when complains occur. The child requires care during the acute stage. Malnourished children suffering from measles need special care. Extra fluids and a soft drink should be given. The patient should be observed for complications and a doctor should be consulted if required.

Prevention and control

Prevention and control of the infection is a practical problem.

1. Isolation of the patients and quarantine of contacts are useful in prevention of infection in susceptible children.
2. Patient should be isolated for several days even after disappearance of rash and symptoms.

The use of measles vaccine for prevention of infection in susceptible children can effectively control the infection. Three vaccines are specified in I.P. 2007 for control of measles.

1. Measles Vaccine (Live): Freeze dried preparation of a suitable attenuated strain of measles virus.
2. Measles and Rubella Vaccine (Live): Freeze dried preparation of suitable attenuated strains of measles virus and rubella virus.
3. Measles, Mumps and Rubella Vaccine (Live): Freeze dried preparation of suitable strains of measles, mumps and rubella virus.

(c) Influenza (Flu)

Influenza is an acute and specific infection of respiratory tract. It is distributed worldwide. It is characterized by abrupt onset with fever, headache, chills, sore throat, cough without much sputum, weakness and severe aches and pains in the back and limbs. Major epidemics occur at intervals of 2-3 years.

Causative organism

It is caused by RNA viruses belonging to the group of myxo viruses – influenza A, B and C strain; para influenza virus types 1, 2 or 3; rhinovirus and adenoviruses.

Incubation period

18 to 72 hours.

Mode of transmission

Source of infection is usually a case or subclinical case. Influenza is spread from person to person mainly by droplet infection or droplet nuclei created by sneezing, coughing or talking. The portal of entry of the virus is the respiratory tract.

Prevention and control

The best approach is prophylactic immunization. A killed vaccine is available but mass immunization before the expected epidemic is difficult. Compulsory notification, isolation and quarantine, especially at ports, are general preventive measures. There is no specific treatment except general supportive measures for upper respiratory infections.

Three vaccines against influenza are included in I.P. 2007:

1. Inactivated Influenza Vaccine (Split virion).
2. Inactivated Influenza Vaccine (Surface antigen).
3. Inactivated Influenza Vaccine (Whole virion).

Treatment

Antiviral drugs particularly neuraminidase inhibitors such as Tamiflu or Relenza have been found effective in treatment of influenza.

(d) Swine flu

In April 2009, a novel flu disease was emerged in Mexico, United States and several other countries. The causative agent of this disease contains genes from all the three flu namely human, pig and bird. Initially it was called as swine flu but later named as influenza A/H1N1.

(e) Diphtheria

It is an acute communicable disease mostly localized in throat, nose and tonsils. It occurs mostly in pre-school children. Adults may be occasionally affected. It is characterized by the involvement of respiratory system and formation of false membrane for a soluble exotoxin. Peculiar inflammation of the surface of membrane to the nose, throat and tonsils occurs. The bacteria also produce toxin, which is absorbed into the blood and causes serious complications in the nervous system and heart.

Causative organism

Diphtheria is caused by *Corynebacterium diphtheria,* a rod shaped Gram positive bacterium. The exotoxin secreted by the bacteria is a powerful poison to man.

Incubation period

2 to 5 days.

Mode of transmission

Diphtheria is spread mainly by droplet infection. It can also be transmitted to susceptible persons directly from infected cutaneous lesions. Diphtheria may also be spread by contaminated objects or foods. The bacteria most commonly infect the nose and throat. The throat infection causes a gray to black, tough, fiber-like covering, which can block the airways. In some cases, diphtheria may first infect the skin, producing skin lesions.

Prevention and control

Most effective preventive measure is artificial active immunization with alum precipitated diphtheria toxoid. The commonly used vaccine is DPT, which protects against three common diseases of the childhood- diphtheria, pertussis and tetanus. Inoculation is done at 1 to 3 months of age and repeated twice at 4 to 6 weeks interval. A booster dose is given at 1.5 years age and then at 5–6 years. During the outbreaks of the disease the following measures are recommended – prompt notification, isolation of the patient at home or in hospital, concurrent and terminal disinfection, and exclusion of contact children from schools for at least 2 weeks.

The following vaccines for prevention of diphtheria are official in I.P. 2007.

1. Adsorbed Diphtheria, Tetanus and Hepatitis B (rDNA) vaccine.
2. Adsorbed Diphtheria, Tetanus and Pertussis (Acellular Component) vaccine and Haemophilus Type b Conjugate Vaccine.
3. Adsorbed Diphtheria, Tetanus and Pertussis (Acellular Component) and Hepatitis B (rDNA) Vaccine.
4. Adsorbed Diphtheria, Tetanus and Pertussis (Acellular Component), Inactivated Poliomyelitis Vaccine and Haemophilus Type b Conjugate Vaccine.
5. Adsorbed Diphtheria, Tetanus, Pertussis (Acellular Component) and Inactivated Poliomyelitis Vaccine.
6. Adsorbed Diphtheria, Tetanus, Pertussis and Poliomyelitis (Inactivated) Vaccine.
7. Adsorbed Diphtheria, Tetanus, Pertussis, Poliomyelitis (Inactivated) and Haemophilus Type b Conjugate Vaccine.
8. Diphtheria and Tetanus Vaccine (Adsorbed).
9. Diphtheria and Tetanus Vaccine (Adsorbed) for Adults and Adolescents.
10. Diphtheria, Tetanus and Pertussis Vaccine (Adsorbed).
11. Diphtheria, Tetanus, Pertussis (Whole Cell), Hepatitis B (rDNA) and Haemophilus Type b Conjugate Vaccine (Adsorbed).
12. Diphtheria, Tetanus, Pertussis (Whole Cell) Hepatitis B (rDNA) Vaccine (Adsorbed).
13. Diphtheria, Tetanus, Pertussis (Whole Cell) and Haemophilus Type b Conjugate Vaccine (Adsorbed).
14. Diphtheria Vaccine (Adsorbed).

Treatment

Treatment should be started immediately. It consists in giving anti-diphtheria serum, antibiotics and relief of symptoms. Acute cases are promptly treated with diphtheria antitoxin doses of 10,000 to 50,000 units. The household and other contacts may be given a prophylactic dose of 500 to 1000 units. One-lack units of penicillin in normal saline can be injected 3 hourly for 2–3 days. Fluid diet should be given till the throat is clear. The patient should be put in bed in absolute rest to minimize complications. People with diphtheria may need to stay in the hospital while the antitoxin is being received.

Other treatments for diphtheria may include:

1. Fluids by IV.
2. Oxygen.

3. Bed rest.
4. Heart monitoring.
5. Insertion of a breathing tube.
6. Correction of airway blockages.

Anyone who has come into contact with the infected person should receive an immunization or booster shots against diphtheria. Protective immunity lasts only 10 years from the time of vaccination, so it is important for adults to get a booster of tetanus-diphtheria (Td) vaccine every 10 years.

(f) Whooping Cough (Pertussis)

Whopping cough is an acute respiratory infection involving the trachea, bronchi and bronchioles. It is very common childhood disease occurring in children under 5 years. The disease develops slowly with fever, cold and an irritating cough. The child then becomes more ill and suffers from the typical cough with the characteristic 'whoop' (loud crowing inspiration). During the coughing phase the child often vomits, the eyes may bulge and there is difficulty in breathing.

Causative organism

Bordetella pertussis or *Haemophillus pertussis* or *Bordetella parapertussis* bacteria.

Incubation period

7–14 days.

Mode of transmission

Whooping cough is spread mainly by droplet infection and direct contact. The main source of infection is nasopharyngeal, laryngeal and bronchial discharges. The germs are present in the nose and throat of the patient and each time an infected person coughs, sneezes or talks, these germs are spread in the air. Most children contact the infection from playmates.

Prevention and control

The best preventive measure is the active immunization of all infants with triple vaccine starting at 1–2 months of age. The general principles of isolation, treatment and disinfection of discharges from the nose and throat are applied for the prevention and control. It is important to protect very young and weak children from exposure. The affected children should be kept away from the school for a period of 6 weeks.

I.P. 2007 recommends the following vaccines for prevention of pertussis:

1. Adsorbed Diphtheria, Tetanus and Pertussis (Acellular Component) vaccine and Haemophilus Type b Conjugate Vaccine.
2. Adsorbed Diphtheria, Tetanus and Pertussis (Acellular Component) and Hepatitis B (rDNA) Vaccine.

3. Adsorbed Diphtheria, Tetanus and Pertussis (Acellular Component), Inactivated Poliomyelitis Vaccine and Haemophilus Type b Conjugate Vaccine.
4. Adsorbed Diphtheria, Tetanus, Pertussis (Acellular Component) and Inactivated Poliomyelitis Vaccine.
5. Adsorbed Diphtheria, Tetanus, Pertussis and Poliomyelitis (Inactivated) Vaccine.
6. Adsorbed Diphtheria, Tetanus, Pertussis, Poliomyelitis (Inactivated) and Haemophilus Type b Conjugate Vaccine.
7. Diphtheria, Tetanus and Pertussis Vaccine (Adsorbed).
8. Diphtheria, Tetanus, Pertussis (Whole Cell), Hepatitis B (rDNA) and Haemophilus Type b Conjugate Vaccine (Adsorbed).
9. Diphtheria, Tetanus, Pertussis (Whole Cell) Hepatitis B (rDNA) Vaccine (Adsorbed)
10. Diphtheria, Tetanus, Pertussis (Whole Cell) and Haemophilus Type b Conjugate Vaccine (Adsorbed).
11. Adsorbed Pertussis Vaccine (Acellular Component).
12. Adsorbed Pertussis Vaccine (Acellular, Co-purified).
13. Pertussis Vaccine.

Treatment

1. Antibiotics such as erythromycin may help in alleviating the symptoms quickly if treatment is started early enough.
2. Unfortunately, in most of the cases whooping cough is diagnosed too late when antibiotics are not very effective. Although, the medicines may help in reducing the patient's ability to spread the disease to others.
3. Infants younger than 18 months need constant supervision because their breathing may temporarily stop during coughing spells.
4. Infants with severe cases should be hospitalized.
5. An oxygen tent with high humidity may be used.
6. Fluids may be given through a vein if coughing spells are severe enough to prevent the person from drinking enough fluids.
7. Sedatives may be prescribed for young children.
8. Cough mixtures, expectorants, and suppressants are usually not helpful and should not be used.

(g) Tuberculosis

Tuberculosis (TB) is a specific communicable disease occurring in acute or chronic form. It primarily affects lungs and causes pulmonary TB; it can also affect intestine, meninges, bones and joints, lymph nodes, skin and other tissues of the body. The disease also affects animals (bovine tuberculosis). TB continues to be major health problem in India. There are about 10 million patients of TB and nearly half a million die of TB every year. Symptoms of the disease usually develop gradually. Cough is the earliest symptom, fever continues for a long time. Pain in the chest, feeling of weakness and loss of weight are associated symptoms. Blood in sputum appears in later stages. In advanced stage of disease, patient develops feeling out of breath on exertion. In children there may only be swelling of the lymph nodes.

Causative organism

Tuberculosis is a contagious disease caused by *Mycobacterium tuberculosis,* which attacks both pulmonary as well as non-pulmonary tissues.

Incubation period

4 to 6 weeks for primary lesions to one year for the disease to develop.

Mode of transmission

Human sources are the open infected cases spreading infection through droplets and vomits. Bovine sources are the milk from infected animals, especially cows. The most common route of transmission is through droplet infection; when a patient coughs, sneezes or talks. Overcrowding, poor ventilation and lighting favor the spread of TB. Flies may act as mechanical carriers.

Prevention and control

General measures are aimed at upliftment of economic status for people to attain high income, decent and sanitary dwellings, reduction of overcrowding, improvement of sanitary conditions both in residential and occupational sites, and most important, high nutritional status. Health education of the people is also very important.

Diagnostic tests

1. Tuberculin skin test.
2. Bronchoscopy.
3. Chest CT scan.
4. Chest X-ray.
5. Interferon-gamma blood test such as the QuantiFERON-TB Gold Test (QFT-G) for TB infection.
6. Sputum examination and cultures.
7. Thoracentesis (insertion of a hollow needle into the pleural cavity through the chest wall in order to withdraw fluid, blood, pus, or air).

Control measures

These are:

1. At the level of the cases suffering (reservoir of infection).
   (a) Early detection of cases through sputum examination for acid-fast bacilli by Ziehl-Neelsen stain and microscopic examination. Chest X-ray investigation is also helpful in detection of TB.
   (b) Treatment and follow up – Treatment must be regular with complete doses of the prescribed drugs for the complete duration, usually 18 months to 2 years. Commonly used drugs are Rifampicin, INH (isoniazid), Streptomycin, Pyrazinaminde, Ethambutol and Thioacetazone.

2. To block the spread of the disease.

(a) Blocking the channels of transmission – while coughing, talking or sneezing the patient should cover his mouth with a piece of cloth, which can be later burnt or reused after boiling.

(b) Sputum should be collected in a wide mouthed container with a lid and disposed of by burning, or collected in a container with phenol and buried.

(c) The patient should sleep in a separate room having good ventilation and direct sunlight. Children should be kept away from the patient. Separate utensils, towels, handkerchiefs etc, should be used by the patient. All family members should be examined and investigated by x-ray and sputum examination.

3. To raise the immunity of non-infected persons.

(a) Immunizing all newborns with BCG vaccine is an important method of TB control. In India BCG vaccination is given to all newborn babies as part of the Expanded Program on Immunization (EPI).

The National Tuberculosis Program (NTP) is in operation since 1962. Its aim is to reduce the problem of TB in the community as quickly as possible to the level where it ceases to be a public health problem.

The District TB program (DTP) is the backbone of the NTP. It is also in operation since 1962.

(b) Cooperative role of voluntary, social welfare organizations, private medical practitioners, TB Association of India etc are important in anti-TB campaign in the country.

Treatment

The first choice drugs used in treatment of tuberculosis are:

1. Isoniazid.
2. Rifampicin.
3. Pyrazinamide.
4. Ethambutol.

Second choice drugs used in treatment of tuberculosis are:

1. Amikacin.
2. Moxifloxacin.
3. Streptomycin.
4. Para-amino salicylic acid.
5. Ethionamide.

It is very important that anti-tubercular drugs are taken according to the prescribed schedule. The infection may become difficult to treat if patient does not take medicine as recommended. The drug may no longer help in treating the infection, if TB bacteria become resistant to treatment.

Recently on 31st Dec 2012 the USFDA has approved Bedaquiline for part treatment of multi-drug resistant tuberculosis (MDR-TB). This drug will be sold under the name Sirturo by Janseen Therapeutics, USA.

INTESTINAL INFECTIONS

(a) Poliomyelitis

Poliomyelitis is an acute, infectious, viral disease affecting the central nervous system and infrequently resulting in paralysis of voluntary muscles of lower extremities. The legs are more affected than arms. It attacks children of all ages especially below 5 years of age. Acute poliomyelitis or infantile paralysis is one of the main crippling diseases of childhood. The attack begins with fever, headache, vomiting, pain and stiffness of the neck, sometimes convulsions followed by paralysis of a limb. Death may occur in rare cases.

Causative organisms

It is caused by poliovirus, which has three distinct serotypes, 1, 2 and 3. Type 1 is most predominant during epidemics. The virus inhabits the alimentary canal and throat of man.

Incubation period

7 to 14 days.

Mode of transmission

It is transmitted usually by the faeco-oral route, through direct contact, and sometimes through milk. The virus multiplies in the throat and intestinal tract and then absorbed and spread through the blood and lymph system. The symptoms of the disease develop after 5 – 35 days (average 7 – 14 days) from the time of infection.

Care of the patient

Unfortunately there is no specific treatment. Complete bed rest preferably in hospital is essential and the affected limb should be supported. To prevent contractures, the limb should be provided passive movements. Physiotherapy to the paralyzed limb is recommended subsequently.

Treatment

Following measures are taken in the treatment of polio.

1. The goal of treatment is to control symptoms while the infection runs its course.
2. People with severe cases may need life-saving measures, especially breathing help.
3. Symptoms are treated based on their severity.
4. Urinary tract infections are treated with antibiotics.
5. Urinary retention is treated with medicines like Bethanechol.
6. Moist heat (heating pads, warm towels) is used to reduce muscle pain and spasms.
7. Painkillers can be used to reduce headache, muscle pain, and spasms.
8. Physical therapy, braces or corrective shoes, or orthopedic surgery to help recover muscle strength and function.

Prevention and control

Following measures are recommended.

1. Notification and isolation of the patient.
2. Proper disposal of urine and faeces. The faeces remain infective for 4 weeks.
3. All sources of water supply should be properly protected and supply of safe and potable drinking water must be ensured.
4. Overcrowding in schools, theatres and other places should be avoided.
5. Active immunization of all children with polio vaccine. Under the Expanded Program on Immunization (EPI), routine administration of three doses of oral polio vaccine is recommended for the age group of 3 to 9 months. A single booster dose is given at the age of 18 months. Hot fluids should be given for half an hour after the vaccine has been administered.
6. Anti-fly measures should be intensified.

Vaccines

Following vaccines are included in I.P. 2007 for prevention of poliomyelitis.

1. Adsorbed Diphtheria, Tetanus and Pertussis (Acellular Component), Inactivated Poliomyelitis Vaccine and Haemophilus Type b Conjugate Vaccine.
2. Adsorbed Diphtheria, Tetanus, Pertussis (Acellular Component) and Inactivated Poliomyelitis Vaccine.
3. Adsorbed Diphtheria, Tetanus, Pertussis and Poliomyelitis (Inactivated) Vaccine.
4. Adsorbed Diphtheria, Tetanus, Pertussis, Poliomyelitis (Inactivated) and Haemophilus Type b Conjugate Vaccine.
5. Poliomyelitis Vaccine (Inactivated).
6. Poliomyelitis Vaccine, Live (Oral).

(b) Hepatitis

Hepatitis is a disease of liver characterized by inflammation of liver cells. The causes of hepatitis may be hepatitis viruses, other infections (toxoplasma, leptospira, Q fever etc), toxins such as alcohol, some industrial organic solvents and plants. The disease may also be autoimmune. Hepatitis A infection (infective hepatitis or epidemic jaundice) is an acute infectious disease characterized by jaundice. It is an endemic disease common in children and young adults all over the world. Epidemics also occur frequently. The onset is accompanied by anorexia followed by progressive jaundice and hepatitis, which may sometimes end in coma and death.

Types of Hepatitis

1. Alcoholic hepatitis.
2. Autoimmune hepatitis.
3. Delta agent (hepatitis D).
4. Drug-induced hepatitis.

5. Hepatitis A.
6. Hepatitis B.
7. Hepatitis C.

Causative organism

Hepatitis is caused by *Hepatitis A virus* found in faeces and blood of infected persons.

Incubation period

2 to 5 weeks.

Mode of transmission

It is spread by the faeco-oral route. The virus is excreted in the stools of the patient. Contamination of water and food may lead to explosive outbreaks. The disease is also spread by direct contact. As a sexually transmitted infection, hepatitis A may occur mainly among homosexual man because of oral-anal contact.

Diagnosis

Physical examination
(a) Enlargement and tenderness of liver.
(b) Fluid in the abdomen (ascites) that can become infected.
(c) Yellowing of the skin.

Laboratory test
(a) Abdominal ultrasound.
(b) Autoimmune blood markers.
(c) Hepatitis virus serologies.
(d) Liver function tests.
(e) Liver biopsy to check for liver damage.
(f) Paracentesis, if fluid is present in abdomen.

Care

There is no specific treatment. The patient must take complete bed rest for 2–3 weeks. A diet rich in fruit juices and glucose is recommended. Fatty foods should be avoided.

Prevention and control

Improvement in sanitation is the only permanent method. During epidemics only boiled water must be used for drinking. Virus is not killed by chlorination of water or other methods of sterilization. Anti-fly measures should be intensified.

Vaccines

Vaccines based on recombinant DNA virus are specified for active immunization against hepatitis in I.P. 2007.

1. Adsorbed Diphtheria, Tetanus and Hepatitis B (rDNA) Vaccine.

2. Adsorbed Diphtheria, Tetanus and Pertussis (Acellular Component) and Hepatitis B (rDNA) Vaccine.
3. Diphtheria, Tetanus, Pertussis (Whole Cell), Hepatitis B (rDNA) and Haemophilus Type b Conjugate Vaccine (Adsorbed).
4. Diphtheria, Tetanus, Pertussis (Whole Cell) Hepatitis B (rDNA) Vaccine (Adsorbed).
5. Hepatitis A (Inactivated) and Hepatitis B (rDNA) Vaccine (Adsorbed).
6. Hepatitis B Vaccine (rDNA).
7. Inactivated Hepatitis A Vaccine (Adsorbed).
8. Inactivated Hepatitis B Vaccine.

(c) Cholera

Cholera is an acute specific infection of the gastro-intestinal tract. It is characterized by sudden onset of severe watery diarrhoea, vomiting resulting in extreme dehydration, low blood pressure and collapse. It occurs in people of all ages and both sexes are affected. It occurs in summer and autumn. Cholera is endemic in Maharashtra, Tamilnadu, Madhya Pradesh, Assam and Andhra Pradesh. Because of excessive loss of fluid and electrolytes the patient becomes rapidly dehydrated. Death may occur if dehydration is not corrected.

Casuative organism

Cholera is caused by *Vibrio cholera,* which are Gram-negative, actively motile, comma shaped bacteria.

Incubation period

Few hours to 5 days.

Mode of transmission

Cholera is spread by faeco-oral route, through ingestion of polluted water or contaminated food. It can also spread through clothes and linen soaked with discharges of infected persons. Flies also spread the infection. Persons attending on cholera patients must wash their hands properly to avoid infecting the food, drink or themselves.

Care of patient

Correction of dehydration is most important. Mild to moderate dehydration can be corrected by oral administration of fluid and electrolytes. In severe dehydration administration of intravenous fluids is necessary.

Oral Rehydration Salts [ORS] consist of sodium chloride – 3.5 g, sodium bicarbonate – 2.5 g, potassium chloride – 1.5 g and glucose – 20 g; dissolved in 1 litre of water.

Prevention and control

Compulsory and prompt notification of cases and isolation of patients, sprinkling of lime water on the floor of patient's room, anti-fly measures, disinfection of patient's excreta and linen are the preventive measures. Cholera vaccine is used for immunization. It contains killed bacteria and is administered subcutaneously in 2 doses of 0.5 mL each at an interval of 4 to 6 weeks.

Treatment

The treatment consists of rehydration and antibiotics. The objective of treatment is to replace fluid and electrolytes lost through diarrhoea. Depending on the condition of patient, fluids may be given by mouth or through a vein (intravenous). The World Health Organization (WHO) has developed an oral rehydration solution that is cheaper and easier to use than the typical intravenous fluid. This solution of sugar and electrolytes is now being used internationally.

Tetracycline and chloramphenicol in doses of 500 mg of either drug 4 times a day is recommended for 3 days. Furalizine and Septran are also recommended as alternative drugs.

National Cholera Control Program is also aimed at gradual elimination of endemic foci by anticipatory preventive measures and surveillance activities for containment of cholera.

(d) Typhoid

Typhoid is an acute communicable disease characterized by a typical continuous fever for 3 to 4 days, relative bradycardia with involvement of lymphoid tissues and considerable constitutional symptoms. Typhoid is usually endemic and occurs throughout the year but frequency of reported cases is higher during rainy season. It is most common in the age group of 6 to 30 years.

Causative organism

Typhoid is caused by the bacillus *Salmonella typhi*.

Incubation period

10 to 15 days.

Mode of transmission

The disease is spread through the faeco-oral route. The bacilli are excreted in the stools and urine of cases and carriers. Indiscriminate defecation and urination leads to spread of infection through soil, water, food and flies. The disease is spread chiefly by ingestion of contaminated food, water, milk and milk products and by consumption of unwashed, raw vegetables. Typhoid can also spread through direct contact, and in a small proportion of cases, through vomits i.e. infected bedclothes, towels etc.

Diagnosis

Widal test is used to diagnose typhoid. It is based on the demonstration of salmonella antibodies against antigens O-somatic and H-flagellar.

Procedure of Widal test
- Patient's serum is doubly diluted by mixing and transferring from 1 : 10 to 1 : 640 in three-four rows. First row usually comprises of Felix tubes,

where somatic *S.* typhi O antigen is added. For all the remaining rows, Dreyer's tubes are taken; where different flagellar H antigens are added. Each tube must contain 0.5 mL of diluted serum. A test tube with only saline is kept in each row as control. All the tubes (including control) in a row are mixed with 0.5 mL of antigen suspension. The first row is treated with *S.* typhi O antigen, the second row with *S.* typhi H antigen, the third row with *S.* paratyphi AH antigen and the fourth row with *S.* paratyphi BH antigen. Since infections by *S.* paratyphi B are rare, this antigen is usually omitted in the test. After all the tubes have been treated with specific antigen suspensions, the Widal rack is placed in a thermostatically controlled water bath maintained at 37ºC for overnight incubation. Another approach is to incubate the tubes at 50–55ºC.

Interpretation of results for Widal test
- The control tubes must be examined first, where they should give no agglutination. The agglutination of O antigen appears as a "matt" or "carpet" at the bottom. Agglutination of H antigens appears loose, wooly or cottony. The highest dilution of serum that produces a positive agglutination is taken as titre. The titres for all the antigens are noted.

Care of patient

The patient requires complete bed rest during the period of fever and for at least 10 to 15 days after the fever comes down; the patient must be given a soft diet as there is ulceration in the small intestine.

Prevention and control

As carriers play an important role in the spread of this infection their prompt detection, isolation and treatment of the suffering patients is very important in controlling outbreaks of typhoid fever. Food should be protected from flies. Raw vegetables and fruits should be taken only after washing them in a weak solution of potassium permanganate. Drinking water and milk must be boiled. Improvement of sanitation especially by ensuring safe and potable water supply, proper excreta disposal etc constitute very useful control measure. TAB vaccine provides protection against typhoid. The vaccine is given in 2 doses of 0.5 mL each subcutaneously at an interval of 4 to 6 weeks. Under the Expanded Program on Immunization (EPI) all children are immunized with TAB vaccine at the time of entry to school.

Vaccines specified in I.P. 2007 for typhoid include the following:
1. Typhoid (Strain Ty 21a) Vaccine, Live (Oral)
2. Typhoid Polysaccharide Vaccine
3. Typhoid Vaccine
4. Typhoid Vaccine (Freeze Dried)

Treatment

In most cases typhoid fever is not fatal hence antibiotics are used in its treatment.

1. Third generation cephalosporins (Ceftrixone, Cefotaxime, Cefixime) are the treatment of choice. Fluoroquinolones such as Ciprofloxacin, Ofloxacin may be used as first choice drug if resistance is uncommon.
2. Ampicillin, Chloramphenicol, Trimethoprim-sulfamethoxazole, Amoxicillin and Ciprofloxacin are also used to treat typhoid.

(e) Food Poisoning

Food poisoning is an acute gastroenteritis acquired through ingestion of contaminated and injurious food or drinks. Poisoning may occur due to living bacteria or their toxins or inorganic chemical substances and poisons derived from plants and animals. It is characterized by history of ingestion of a common food, attack of many persons at the same time, and similarity of symptoms and signs in majority cases.

Causative agent

Bacterial food poisoning is caused by the ingestion of foods contaminated by living bacteria or their toxins.

Non-bacterial food poisoning is caused by chemicals such as arsenic, tin, copper sulfate, fluorides, pesticides, fertilizers, injurious preservatives, additives and adulterants. Use of cheap enamel-ware in which acidic foods dissolve antimony, is usually responsible for food poisoning.

1. Salmonellosis

It is caused by *Salmonella typhimurium, Salmonella entericides* and *Salmonella cholersuis*. The infection spreads through contaminated meat, milk and milk products, sausages, custards, eggs and egg products. Infected rats and mice may also contaminate foodstuffs by their faeces and urine.

Incubation period: 10 to 24 hours.

The causative organism multiplies in the intestine causing acute enteritis and colitis. The onset is sudden with chills, fever, nausea, vomiting and a profuse watery diarrhea lasting for 2-3 days.

2. Staphylococcal food poisoning

It is caused by enterotoxins of *Staphylococcus aureus*. Salads, custards, milk and milk products contaminated with staphylococcus are responsible for poisoning.

Incubation period: 1 to 6 hours. Poisoning occurs from ingestion of toxins by bacteria in the contaminated food. The toxins act directly on the intestine and CNS. Fever is rare.

3. Botulism

It is caused by exotoxin of *Clostridium botulinum* usually found in under-processed foods. The organism is widely distributed in soil, dust and the intestinal tract of animals. It enters the food as spores. Home preserved foods, smoked or pickled fish, home-made cheese and similar low acid foods are chief sources of botulism.

Incubation period: 12 to 36 hours.

Symptoms

Botulism is characterized by dyspepsia, diplopia, ptosis, dysarthria, blurring of vision, muscle weakness etc. Fever is generally absent. The toxin being thermolabile, food can be rendered safe by heating at 100°C for a few minutes before use. Antitoxin acts as prophylactic against botulism. Active immunization with botulism toxoid is a preventive measure. Guanidine HCl, 15 to 40mg/kg body weight can be given orally. *Clostridium welchi*, an anaerobic organism also causes mild symptoms.

Prevention and control

Prevention of bacterial and chemical contamination of foods is most important. This can be achieved through hygienic food handling and use of clean utensils. Refrigeration of raw and processed food is also useful. Foods should be prepared at adequate temperatures in clean utensils. It should be kept covered to avoid access to rats, mice, flies and dust. Contaminated meat being a source of infection, the food animals must be free from infection. The examination of animals before and after slaughter by veterinary staff is yet another preventive measure. Strict supervision of restaurants, canteens, messes etc in respect of food quality and hygienic cooking methods must be practiced. Over and above these measures, health education particularly for food handlers and their personal hygiene are necessary for effective control of food poisoning.

(f) Hookworm Infestation

A hookworm is a nematode, which lives in the small intestine as a parasite. The eggs are excreted in the stools and develop into larvae in a warm moist soil. Whenever in contact with human skin they penetrate it and are carried to lungs, go up the air passages and windpipe and finally swallowed. Further development takes place in the small intestine. Two species of hookworms i.e. *Ancylostoma duodenale* and *Necator americanus* commonly infect humans. The infection of *A. duodenale* is common in Europe, Egypt and India (Assam, West Bengal, Bihar, Orissa, Andhra Pradesh, Tamil Nadu, Karnataka, Kerala and Maharashtra) whereas *N. americanus* predominates in America, Sub-Saharan Africa, Southest Asia, Indonesia and China. Hookworms are thought to infect more than 600 million people in the world including 45 million people that suffer from ancyclostomiasis in India. Hookworm infestation causes severe anemia, joint pains, dyspepsia, oedema and eosinophelia. This results in lowered body resistance, retarded development in children, mental retardation and loss of efficiency in infested persons.

Causative agent

Ancyclostoma duodenale and *Necator americanus*.

Incubation period

Eggs appear in the stools about 6 weeks after penetration of the skin by larvae.

Mode of transmission

The infection is acquired through the skin. When a person walks about barefoot in soil contaminated with the stools of a hookworm patient, the infective larvae penetrates through the skin of the feet.

Prevention and control

The affected persons must be treated with Alcopar (bephenium hydroxy naphthoate) and tetrachloro ethylene. Proper disposal of excreta by the construction and use of sanitary latrines is essential to prevent the pollution of soil due to eggs excreted in the stools of the patients. Health education of the people emphasizing the importance of wearing shoes and not walking barefoot is recommended as a personal preventive measure. Fresh stool should not be used as manure rather it should be composted.

Treatment

1. Benzimidazoles (Albendazole and Mebendazole) are the most common treatment for hookworm infestation. Benzimidazoles act by binding to the nematode's β-tubulin and subsequently inhibiting microtubule poly-merization within the parasite.
2. In certain circumstances, Levamisole and Pyrantel pamoate may be used.
3. WHO also recommends anthelmintic treatment in pregnant women after the first trimester. It is recommended that if the patient also suffers from anemia then Ferrous sulfate (200 mg) be administered three times daily at the same time as anthelmintic treatment; this should be continued until hemoglobin values return to normal, which could take up to 3 months.

ARTHROPOD-BORNE INFECTIONS

(a) Plague

Plague is a highly infectious disease transmitted to man by infected rat flea. It is primarily a disease of animals (zoonotic disease). Man is affected incidentally. Plague affects people of all ages and both sexes. It is characterized by high fever, inflammation of lymphatic glands, forming buboes and sometimes by pneumonia or septicemia. The lymph nodes swell rapidly to the size of a hen's egg or larger. They are painful and are called *buboes*. Sometimes the lungs may be affected and there is high fever with rigor, headache, bodyache, cough with expectoration and pain in chest. The patient suffers from breathlessness. The disease is notorious for long silence followed by sudden reappearance. In India not a single case was reported since 1966 but in 1994 there was an outbreak of human plague in Surat.

Human plague is of three varieties:

1. *Bubonic plague*: It is the most common form and occurs through rat fleas. There is fever, prostration with inflammation of regional lymph glands commonly those in groin, axilla and neck, when buboes are formed.
2. *Pneumonic plague*: It is spread by droplet infection from man to man and does not spread through rat fleas. It is usually fatal.

3. *Septicemia plague*: The blood infection occurs without the formation of buboes. It is rare but usually fatal.

Casuative organism

Plague is caused by *Pasturella pestis,* a Gram-negative, non-motile, coccobacillus, which is present in buboes of all cases of bubonic plague, in sputum of pneumonic variety and in blood of septicemia cases.

Incubation period

Bubonic plague – 3 to 6 days; Pneumonic plague – 1 to 4 days.

Mode of transmission

Plague is transmitted to man mainly through the rat flea, which acts as a vector and transmits the disease from infected rodents. The infected rat flea transmits the disease mainly through bites. Pneumonic plague is transmitted from the case to new host *through droplet infection.*

Sources of infection are the infected rats and other rodents, which exist as natural foci.

Prevention and control

The following measures are recommended:

1. Early diagnosis and case detection.
2. Compulsory notification, isolation of cases and prompt treatment.
3. Infected place should be evacuated and arrangements made for disinfection of the house and rat destruction campaign. Persons from infected house should be segregated.

During an outbreak of plague, mass vaccination should be done. Killed plague vaccine is given subcutaneously in two doses at an interval of 1 to 2 weeks. In case of emergency, a single dose of the vaccine should be given.

All contacts and those exposed to the risk of infection are given Tetracycline or Sulfonamides for a week, as a prophylactic measure. Rodenticides e.g. Barium Carbonate, Zinc Phosphide can be used to control rodents. Wire cage traps are generally used for trapping the rats. Improvement of general sanitation and housing is the only long term measure of control.

Anti-rat campaign has main emphasis on:
(i) preventing access of rats to food supply, and
(ii) destruction of rats.

Sputum, discharges from lymph nodes and articles used by the patient must be disinfected. Dead bodies must be handled aseptically.

Lay public should be educated about the anti-plague measures by lecture, hand bills, films and slides to show how infection occurs and to teach them how to guard against rats and fleas.

Treatment

1. People infected with plague need immediate treatment. If treatment is not received within 24 hours when the first symptoms appear, death may occur.

2. Antibiotics such as Streptomycin, Gentamicin, Doxycycline, or Ciprofloxacin are used to treat plague.
3. Oxygen, intravenous fluids, and respiratory support usually are also needed.

(b) Malaria

Malaria is a protozoal infection. It is one of the most important health problems in India. The entire population is deemed to be under malarial risk. People of all ages and both sexes are affected by malaria. There is no natural immunity and practically all races are susceptible except the Negroes who are immune.

Malaria is characterized by:

1. *Cold stage* i.e. sudden onset of fever with sensation of extreme cold, lasting for 15 to 60 minutes.
2. *Hot stage* i.e. temperature shooting up to 106°C, patient feeling burning hot and intense headache.
3. *Sweating stage* i.e. profuse sweating and fall in temperature, lasting from 2 to 6 hours.

If the infection persists, gradual anemia develops and the liver and spleen are enlarged. Typical attacks of malaria fever may not be observed sometimes due to maturation of generations of the parasite at different times. The attacks occur regularly every alternate day or every fourth day. The patient is free from the symptoms in between the attacks.

Causative organism

It is caused by the malarial parasites (Plasmodium) of the following types: *Plasmodium vivax, P. falciparum, P. malariae,* and *P. ovale.*

Incubation period

10 to 30 days.

Mode of transmission

Malaria is mainly transmitted through the bite of infected *Anopheles* mosquitoes. Mosquitoes become infected after feeding on a person harboring malarial parasites in the blood. The sexual cycle of the parasite takes place in the mosquito and the parasite develops into the infective stages (sporozoites) within 2–3 weeks. The sporozoites are injected in the new susceptible host when the mosquito feeds on him. After circulating for a short time in the blood of the human being the parasites enter the liver and develop into form, which are able to invade the red blood cells and develop into gametes. This completes the asexual cycle of the parasite. The mosquito feeding on the man sucks the gametes and thus the cycle of transmission continues.

Sometimes malaria is also transmitted through transfusion of blood containing malarial parasites. Congenital malaria (infection of the newborn from an infected mother) is relatively rare.

Prevention and control

WHO has recommended the following anti-malarial measures:

Measures to be applied by individuals	Measures to be applied by community
Prevention of man/vector contact using mosquito repellants, protective clothing, bed nets, screening of houses.	Prevention of man/vector contact through selection of proper site and screening of houses.
Destruction of adult mosquitoes through the use of domestic insecticidal sprays including aerosols.	Destruction of adult mosquitoes through insecticidal sprays.
Destruction of mosquito larvae.	Destruction of mosquito larvae.
Source reduction of mosquitoes like filling small scale drains, etc.	Source reduction through effective sanitation, water management and drainage schemes.
Chemoprophylaxis and chemotherapy against malaria parasite.	Measures against malaria parasites such as presumptive treatment, radical treatment and mass drug treatment.

Community participation and health education are very important for any successful malaria control campaign.

National Malaria Eradication Program was initiated in 1968 and a modified operation plan was started in 1977.

Attempts to develop anti-malarial vaccine are going on in India and abroad.

Treatment

1. Malaria (particularly Falciparum malaria) is a medical emergency that requires a hospital stay. The choice of medication depends in part on where the patient is infected.
2. Chloroquine is often used as an anti-malarial medication, though chloroquine-resistant infections are common in some parts of the world.
3. Chloroquine-resistant infections are treated by following drugs:
   (a) Combination of Quinidine or Quinine + Doxycycline/Tetracycline/Clindamycin.
   (b) Atovaquone plus Proguanil (Malarone).
   (c) Mefloquine or Artesunate.
   (d) Combination of Pyrimethamine + Sulfadoxine (Fansidar).
4. Medical care, including fluids through a vein (IV) and other medications and breathing (respiratory) support may be needed.

(c) Filariasis

It is a major public health problem in India. It is endemic all over India except in Jammu & Kashmir. It is a communicable disease transmitted through mosquito bites. Filariasis mainly affects the lymphatic system. Heavily infected areas exist in Uttar Pradesh, Bihar, Andhra Pradesh, Orissa, Tamil Nadu, Kerala and Gujarat. People of all ages and both sexes are susceptible. Filariasis is not fatal but it disables and deforms a person especially due to swelling of the legs and the external genitalia, a condition called *elephantitis*.

Casusative organism

Filariasis is caused by two nematode worms – W*ucherria bancrofti* and *Wucherria malayi*. These parasites are long, thread-like worms with tapering ends, easily visible with naked eyes.

Mode of transmission

The disease is transmitted from an infected person to a new host through the bite of a mosquito. The main vectors are *Culex fatigans* and *Mansonides mosquitoes.*

Prevention and control

Anti-mosquito measures and protection from mosquito bites are most important. Diethylcarbamazine (*Hetran*) is the only drug available against filariasis. The drug should be given in doses of 6 mg/kg-body weight per day orally for 12 days, preferably in divided doses, after meals.

National Filariasis Control Program was started in 1955 but in 1978 its operational components have been merged with Urban Malaria Scheme.

Adult mosquito control (vector control) can be achieved by insecticidal spray, larvicidal measures, removal of aquatic plants and improvement of environmental sanitation. Health education of the people is most important in dealing with the problem of Filariasis.

Treatment

1. Albendazole (a broad-spectrum anthelmintic) combined with Ivermectin is the treatment of choice.
2. Combination of Diethylcarbamazine (DEC) and Albendazole is also effective.

All of these treatments are *micro*filaricides; they have no effect on the adult worms.

SURFACE INFECTIONS

(a) Rabies (Hydrophobia)

Rabies is the only communicable disease of man, which is almost always fatal. It is an acute viral infectious disease of the nervous system transmitted by the bite of a rabid animal, commonly dogs. In affected man the most important characteristic is hydrophobia or 'fear of water'. *There is no treatment of hydrophobia.*

Causative organism

Rabies is caused by neurotropic RNA virus of rhabdovirus group. It is found in saliva, urine, lymph, blood, milk of infected animals, and multiplies in nerve cells. The size of the virus is 100 to 150 millimicrons.

Incubation period

10 days to 8 months depending on the site and severity of the bite by the rabid animal.

Mode of transmission

Rabies is primarily a zoonotic disease. Wild animals like foxes, jackals, wolves and mongooses are the reservoirs of rabies virus. These wild animals transmit the infection to domestic animals like dogs. The urban cycle is maintained by the stray dog population, which is responsible for 99% of human infection. The disease is usually transmitted by the bite of a rabid animal but man may contact the infection by contamination of injured skin by the saliva of a rabid animal. Thus saliva is the main source of infection.

Care of patient

The hydrophobia patient should be isolated. Care and treatment should be aimed at minimizing the suffering of the patient and protecting the persons attending the patient. Patient should be kept in a dark and quiet room, undisturbed, protected from exposure to cold droughts or other stimuli likely to precipitate spasms or convulsions. Morphine should be given freely for sedation or convulsions. A person attending the patient should wear gloves, boots and gowns to protect himself from contact with the patient's saliva.

Prevention and control

The wound caused by the bite by rabid animal should be washed with soap and water, dried and cauterized with carbolic acid, permanganate crystals or pure nitric acid. The tissue beneath the bite should be infiltrated with 5 mL of anti-rabies hyper-immune serum. Wound must not be sutured.

Pasteur's Prophylactic Treatment utilizes anti-rabies vaccine (ARV). The treatment is given immediately if animal is clinically rabid or was killed without examination or escaped and if wound is contaminated with fresh saliva. If possible, the animal should be observed for 10 days because within this time rabies would develop if the animal was infected.

Anti-rabies vaccine is a nerve tissue vaccine prepared from the brain of adult sheep or goat and inactivated by phenol. BPL vaccine is β-propiolactone inactivated duck embryo vaccine. Recently human diploid cell tissue culture vaccine (HDCV) inactivated by BPL is also available, which is best post-exposure anti-rabies vaccine. Six subcutaneous injections of 0.1mL are given on the day of the bite and then on 3rd, 7th, 14th, 30th and 90th day. Rhesus cell strain rabies vaccine (RDRV) is given in 5 injections. For post-exposure therapy along with anti-rabies vaccine, human anti-rabies globulin (IgA) is also administered in dose of 20 IU/kg body weight as single intramuscular injection. Control of rabies in dogs requires destruction of all stray dogs, registration and immunization of pet dogs and educating the public about rabies and its prevention.

(b) Trachoma

Trachoma is an infectious disease of the eyes characterized by inflammation of the conjunctiva and cornea. It is one of the main causes of blindness in India. It is especially prevalent in the States of Punjab, Rajasthan and Uttar Pradesh.

Causative organism

Trachoma is caused by *Chlamydiae trachomatis,* which invades mucous membrane covering the surface of the eye ball and lining of the lids.

Incubation period

5 to 12 days.

Mode of transmission

Eye to eye transmission is the rule. It spreads by direct or indirect contact with ocular discharges of infected persons or vomits e.g. infected fingers, towels, *kajal* or *surma,* handkerchiefs. Flies carrying eye discharges from the infected person can transmit the infection to a healthy person. The spread of trachoma is favored by malnutrition, overcrowding and inadequate personal cleanliness.

Prevention and control

Contributory factors like personal hygiene, socio-economic conditions and overall living conditions must be improved.

Sulphacetamide eye drops (10–20%) and Tetracycline eye ointments are used in the treatment of trachoma. For mass treatment Tetracycline eye ointment (1%) b.i.d. for 5 consecutive days in a month for 6 months is recommended. Erythromycin and Rifamycin have also been used in the treatment of trachoma. Trachoma treatment can be given to the entire community (mass treatment or blanket treatment). All children under 10 years age should be given blanket treatment. Health education of the people about the mode of transmission of the disease and its prevention are other preventive measures. National Trachoma Control Program was started in 1963, which is now integrated with National Program in Prevention and Control of Visual Impairments and Blindness.

Treatment

1. If used in initial stage, antibiotics (Doxycycline and Erythromycin) can prevent long-term complications.
2. In certain cases, eyelid surgery may be needed to prevent long-term scarring, which can lead to blindness, if not corrected.

(c) Tetanus

Tetanus is an acute disease characterized by painful spasms and twitching of the jaw muscles. This causes difficulty in opening of the mouth and in mastication (lock jaws). Contraction of the muscles of the neck and trunk makes the neck rigid and the body arched characteristically likes a bow. It is an important endemic infection in India. It is also an important cause of infant mortality. It can also affect older children and adults. The disease is very widely distributed in rural areas.

Causative agent

Tetanus is caused by the endotoxin of *Clostridium tetani*.

Incubation period

3 to 21 days.

Mode of transmission

The tetanus bacilli are found in the intestinal tract of horses and cattle. Spread is always through injury and invasion through which the contaminated matter with tetanus spores makes its entry.

Prevention and control

All wounds should be thoroughly cleaned and 3% Iodine solution should be applied. General hygienic conditions of the people must be improved. Tetanus is entirely preventable by active immunization with tetanus toxoid. Children under 5 years age are routinely protected with triple vaccine (Diphtheria, Pertussis and Tetanus).

Passive immunization is carried out with Anti Tetanus Serum (ATS) or Human Tetanus Immunoglobulinin in non-immune cases and for immediate protection of the persons after trachoma. Penicillin and Tetracycline are also given to the injured persons as these antibiotics kill the tetanus bacilli.

Following vaccines are included in I.P. 2007 for active immunization against tetanus:

1. Adsorbed Diphtheria, Tetanus and Hepatitis B (rDNA) Vaccine.
2. Adsorbed Diphtheria, Tetanus and Pertussis (Acellular Component) and Haemophilus Type B Conjugate Vaccine.
3. Adsorbed Diphtheria, Tetanus and Pertussis (Acellular Component) and Hepatitis B (rDNA) Vaccine.
4. Adsorbed Diphtheria, Tetanus and Pertussis (Acellular Component), Inactivated Poliomyelitis Vaccine and Haemophilus Type B Conjugate Vaccine.
5. Adsorbed Diphtheria, Tetanus, Pertussis (Acellular Component) and Inactivated Poliomyelitis Vaccine.
6. Adsorbed Diphtheria, Tetanus, Pertussis and Poliomyelitis (Inactivated) Vaccine.
7. Adsorbed Diphtheria, Tetanus, Pertussis, Poliomyelitis (Inactivated) and Haemophilus Type b Conjugate Vaccine.

(d) Leprosy

Leprosy (Hansen's disease) is a chronic infectious disease characterized by lesions of the skin and by involvement of peripheral nerves with consequent anaesthesia, muscle weakness, paralysis and trophic changes in the skin, muscles and small bones of hands and feet. In chronic cases, deformities such as claw hands, claw fingers, wrist drop, foot drop, facial paralysis, disfigurement of ears and shortening of fingers and toes etc may be present. It is probably the oldest disease known to the mankind. All ages are prone to infection although it mainly affects children and young adults. It is a major public health problem and is widespread in most parts of the country. The states of Tamil Nadu and Andhra Pradesh are particularly severely affected.

Causative organism

Leprosy is caused by *Mycobacterium leprae,* an acid-fast bacillus discovered by Dr. Hansen (hence the name).

Incubation period

6 months to 8 years.

Types of leprosy

There are two types of leprosy:

1. *Non-lepromatous* type in which there is good resistance of the body and hence lesions are localized.
2. *Lepromatous* type in which there is poor resistance of the body with the result that the lepra bacilli multiply and the lesions are generalized.

Mode of transmission

A case of leprosy is only known source of the disease. It is mainly transmitted by continuous, prolonged contact with an infected person. Droplet infection and fomites don't play an important role. The role of insects in the transmission of the infection is suspected but not established. Bacilli may also be transmitted via breast milk from lepromatous mothers or tattooing needles.

Prevention and control

The main principles of leprosy control are early diagnosis and complete treatment to render the patient non-infectious. Early recognition of the disease and its notification and isolation of infectious cases are general preventive measures.

Lepers (leprosy patients) can be kept in leprosarium, hospitals or leper homes.

The National Leprosy Control Program (NLCP) was launched in 1954-55. Under this program, urban leprosy centers, leprosy hospitals, wards and reconstructive surgery units have been established.

Leprosy is not a hereditary disease and is curable.

Treatment

Chemotherapy is of vital importance in the control of leprosy. Following antibiotics are used in the treatment of leprosy:

1. Dapsone (DDS)
2. Rifampicin
3. Clofazimine
4. Fluoroquinolines
5. Macrolides
6. Minocycline

Generally more than one antibiotic are given together. Penicillin and Streptomycin are of particular value for the control of secondary infections. Aspirin (NSAID), Prednisone (corticosteroid) are used to control inflammation.

SEXUALLY-TRANSMITTED DISEASES

(a) Syphilis

Syphilis is a sexually transmitted disease (STD). It is not only a medical problem but also a social and psychological one. The disease may ultimately result in serious complications such as enlargement of the heart and blood vessels, blindness, deafness, paralysis, insanity and sterility.

Causative organism

Syphilis is caused by *Trepenoma pallidum,* a spiral shaped bacterium, which passes through cracks in skin or mucous membrane. The entry occurs directly during sexual intercourse or congenitally by fetus in uterus.

Incubation period

The incubation period of syphilis varies from 9 to 90 days.

Mode of spread

An infected person like a prostitute is the source of infection. The disease is spread directly through sexual intercourse with an infected person or indirectly through transfusion of blood from an infected person and through the placenta. A single infected person can serve as the source of infection to several healthy persons. All the factors that perpetuate prostitution; such as sexual dissatisfaction, divorces, rapid industrialization and tendency to consider prostitution as easy method of earning money; favor the transmission of sexually transmitted diseases like syphilis.

Prevention and control

Case finding is of primary importance in reducing the source of infection. For treatment of syphilis the drug of choice is long-acting Penicillin. Follow up treatment in syphilis consists of i) every month for first six months, ii) every 3 months for next 6 months, and iii) subsequently every 6 months for a period of 2 years.

Treatment

1. A single dose of intramuscular Penicillin G or a single dose of oral Azithromycin is the first choice treatment for uncomplicated syphilis.
2. Third generation Cephalosporin antibiotic Ceftriaxone is equally effective as penicillin.
3. If a person is allergic to penicillin, Ceftriaxone may be used.
4. Doxycycline and Tetracycline are the alternative choice for treatment of early infections of syphilis (not recommended during pregnancy due to risk of birth defects).
5. For the treatment of neurosyphilis large doses of intravenous Penicillin is given for a minimum of 10 days due to poor penetration of Penicillin G into the central nervous system.

(b) Gonorrhea

Gonorrhea is an acute infectious venereal disease characterized by inflammation of the urethra, painful micturition, purulent discharge and liability to certain complications such as ophthalmia, endocarditis, and arthritis. It is more prevalent than syphilis. About 150 million more patients of gonorrhea are added every year.

Causative organism

It is caused by *Neisseria gonorrhoeae,* a Gram-negative intracellular diplococcus.

Incubation period

2 days to 2 weeks.

Mode of transmission

The disease spreads from the infected to the healthy partner mainly through sexual intercourse. During delivery, the eyes of a baby can be infected from a mother suffering from gonorrhea, resulting in gonococcal conjunctivitis of the newborn. In rare cases it may be caused indirectly by infected towels, bedclothes etc.

Prevention and control

Health education of the people is important.

Treatment

There are two goals in treatment of gonorrhea; the first is to cure the infection in the patient, and the second is to locate and test all of the other people with whom the person had sexual contact, and treat them to prevent further spread of the disease.

WHO recommends the following regimen of treatment for gonorrhea:
(i) aqueous Benzyl penicillin sodium, 5 million units plus 1 to 2 g Probenecid;
(ii) aqueous Procaine penicillin, 4 to 8 million units plus 1 to 2 g Probenecid; and (iii) Ampicillin 3 to 5 g single dose plus 1 to 2 g Probenecid.

Septran and Kanamycin are also used in the treatment. Follow up is recommeded on 7th, 14th, 21st and 28th day.

(c) Acquired Immune Deficiency Syndrome (AIDS)

Acquired Immune Deficiency Syndrome (AIDS) was first detected in U.S.A. amongst homosexuals in 1979. It is caused by a virus called HIV (Human Immunodeficiency Virus). It destroys the immune system in the body (the body gradually becomes unable to fight infection). According to WHO more than 25 million people have died of AIDS around the world since its detection and more than 33 million people are living with AIDS worldwide.

Symptoms

People infected with HIV may take 10 years or more to develop symptoms. This period is known as asymptomatic HIV infection, which is followed by early symptomatic HIV infection and later advanced to AIDS in which CD4 T cell count is under 200 cells/mm^3.

Because of damaged immune system, people infected with AIDS are susceptible to infections, which normally do not develop in healthy individuals. Some common symptoms of AIDS are: chills, fever, sweats (particularly at night), swollen lymph glands, weakness, and weight loss.

Opportunistic infections

In AIDS active immunity of patient is damaged due to destruction of CD4 T cells (cells of immune system known as helper cells) hence they are prone to the infection, which normally do not occur in healthy individuals. These are known as opportunistic infections.

List of diseases associated with AIDS according to the CD4 T cells count

CD4 T cell count	Common illness
1. < 350 cells/mm^3	Herpes simplex virus; Herpes zoster; Kaposi's sarcoma; Non-Hodgkin's lymphoma; Tuberculosis; Oral or vaginal due to *Candida albicans* infection.
2. < 200 cells/mm^3	Bacillary angiomatosis (caused by bacteria *Bartonella*); *Candida esophagitis*; *Pneumocystis carinii* pneumonia (now called as *Pneumocystis jiroveci* pneumonia)
3. < 100 cells/mm^3	AIDS dementia; *Cryptococcal meningitis*; *Cryptosporidium diarrhoea*; Leukoencephalopathy; Toxoplasma encephalitis (*Toxoplasma gondii*); Wasting syndrome (caused by HIV)
4. < 50 cells/mm^3	Cytomegalovirus infection; Mycobacterium avium complex

Causative organism

It is caused by Human immunodeficiency virus (HIV). When HIV enters a person's body, it destroys certain immune cells, which normally help the body protect itself from diseases. Hence it makes the body vulnerable to a variety of life-threatening infections and cancers.

Mode of transmission

The virus is transmitted via blood and other body fluids. Anal intercourse is the commonest cause. Next to homosexuals are habitual IV drug abusers. Prostitutes infected by the males suffering from AIDS can also spread disease to others. Pregnant females suffering from disease can pass it onto unborn children. In an HIV infected person, the sexual fluids i.e. semen or vaginal fluids, contain the virus. HIV is therefore transmitted through unprotected sexual intercourse with an HIV infected person. Use of HIV blood contaminated needles or syringes can also transmit HIV from one person to another. HIV *infection is not transmitted through casual everyday contact like shaking hands, touching, hugging, kissing, coughing, sneezing, using the same telephone instrument, swimming pool or toilet seat, sharing eating utensils or foods, bites of mosquitoes and other insects. Donating blood is safe.*

Diagnosis and monitoring

Following tests are used for diagnosis of AIDS and monitoring of AIDS patients:

1. Enzyme linked immunosorbent assay (ELISA).
2. Radio immunoassay (RIA).
3. CD4 cell count.
4. HIV RNA level (viral load).

Incubation period

It varies from 6 months to 10 years. The disease is common in 15 to 50 years age group. 60% of infected persons die within one year and 80 to 90% within two years. About 10 million persons are affected by AIDS in the world.

Prevention and control

Safe sex is the most important preventive measure. Always a pre-lubricated condom should be used throughout sexual intercourse if any partner is suspected to be infected with HIV. A condom should never be re-used and properly disposed. The blood should be tested for HIV prior to transfusion. Safe blood is certified and stamped on the label as follows: *HIV, HBS Antigen, VDRL negative.* All needles and syringes used in blood transfusion should be properly sterilized and, to avoid any risk, sterilized disposable needles and syringes must be used. A woman who is a carrier of HIV should avoid pregnancy.

The Government of India has launched a national plan of action to prevent and control the spread of AIDS in the country.

Pharmacists can play a vital role in educating the general public about AIDS and its prevention.

Treatment

Presently, there is no treatment which can provide cure for AIDS, but quality of life can be improved in patients by antiretroviral therapy, which suppresses virus replication. There are currently more than 20 approved *antiretroviral drugs* in the US and Europe (including combined formulations) and many more in the expanded access programmes and trials.

Most antiretroviral drugs have at least three names. Sometimes a drug is referred to by its research or chemical name, such as AZT. The second name is the generic name for all drugs with the same chemical structure; for example AZT is also known as Zidovudine. The third name is the brand name given by the pharmaceutical company; one of the brand names for Zidovudine is Retrovir. Lastly, an abbreviation of the common name might sometimes also be used, such as ZDV, which is the fourth name given to Zidovudine.

Highly active antiretroviral therapy (HAART) is combination of some different class of antiretroviral drugs, which may be very effective in reducing the number of HIV virus. It improves the T-cell counts and helps immune system to recover from HIV infection. HAART does not provide cure from AIDS, instead it just increases the survival period of patients and has been proved very effective in increasing the lifetime of patients suffering from AIDS.

Three main classes of antiretroviral drugs used in various combinations under HAART are:

1. Nucleoside analogue reverse transcriptase inhibitors (NRITIs).
2. Non-nucleoside reverse transcriptase inhibitors (NNRTIs).
3. Protease inhibitors (PIs).

8

Non-Communicable Diseases

INTRODUCTION

Diseases which are non-infectious are grouped as non-communicable diseases or NCDs. The World Health Organization has reported the NCDs as the leading cause of death in the world. About 35 and 36 million people died from NCDs in the year 2005 and 2008, respectively. NCDs are estimated to account for 53% of all deaths in India.

The characteristics of non-communicable diseases are (i) long duration, and (ii) slow progression.

Diseases included in NCD are discussed below:

CANCER

Next to cardiovascular disease, cancer constitutes the second leading causes of mortality in developed countries. It is one of the 10 leading causes of death in India and its rank is advancing year to year. Over 5 lakh new cases of cancer and 3 lakh deaths are estimated in the country every year. Out of an estimated total of 50 million deaths annually in the world, more than 5 million deaths are due to cancer.

Cancer (malignancy) can be regarded as a group of diseases characterized by an abnormal growth of cells, ability to invade adjacent tissues and even distant organs; and finally the death of the affected patient if the tumor has prolonged beyond that stage when it can be successfully removed. The increasing number of cases of cancer is due to the aging population, environment changes, and better diagnostic facilities.

Cancer can occur at any site of the body and may involve any type of the cells.

Etiology

The etiology of cancer is not exactly understood. Basically it is a disease of the cells. The contributing agents leading to cancer vary in different types of cancers. Such external agents are known as carcinogens. A **carcinogen** may be defined as an agent or substance that can transform normal cells into nepotistic ones.

Tumor and cancer

A mass of tissue formed as a result of abnormal, excessive, uncoordinated, autonomous and purposeless proliferation of cells is called **tumor**. Tumors may be of two types:

1. *Benign:* Slow-growing and localized without causing much difficulty to host.
2. *Malignant:* Proliferates rapidly, spreads throughout the body and may eventually cause death of the host; commonly termed as cancer.

Causes of cancer

(a) Environmental factors

Tobacco smoking/chewing is largely responsible for the cancer of lungs, larynx, mouth, pharynx, oesophagus, bladder, pancreas and probably kidney. Excessive use of alcoholic beverages is associated with oesophageal and liver cancer. Dietary factors are also related to cancer e.g. smoked fish – stomach cancer, dietary fibers – intestinal cancer, beef consumption – bowel cancer, high fat diet – breast cancer. Occupational exposure to benzene, arsenic, cadmium, chromium, vinyl chloride, asbestos, polyacrylic hydrocarbons may lead to cancer. Some viruses are also suspected to be carcinogenic. Parasitic infection may increase the risk of cancer e.g. schistosomiasis may result into carcinoma of the bladder. Other factors include sunlight, radiation, air and water pollution, medication (e.g. estrogens) and pesticides. Some customs, habits and life-styles are also related to cancer e.g. smoking – lung cancer, tobacco and betel chewing – oral cancer etc.

(b) Genetic factors

These are less conspicuous and more difficult to identify e.g. retinoblastoma occurs in children of the same parent. Mongols are more likely to develop leukemia than normal children.

Symptoms

Although symptoms of cancer depend on the type and location of cancer yet following symptoms occur commonly with most cancers:

1. Chills
2. Fatigue
3. Fever
4. Loss of appetite

5. Malaise
6. Night sweats
7. Weight loss.

Diagnosis

Cancer is most frequently diagnosed by following techniques:
1. Blood tests for detecting chemicals such as tumor markers.
2. Biopsy of tumor.
3. Bone marrow biopsy for lymphoma or leukemia.
4. Chest X-ray
5. Complete blood count (CBC).
6. Computed Tomography (CT) scan.
7. Magnetic Resonance Imaging (MRI).

Prevention and control

1. Environmental measures have to be taken, for example in case of chemical carcinogens.
2. Ways of life have to be changed, for example giving up the habit of tobacco chewing, cigarette smoking, improving genital hygiene etc.
3. Early diagnosis and surgical removal have to be implemented, for example in breast cancer, mass surveys and screening might be useful, especially in old people.
4. Cancer detection techniques, for example exfoliate cytology and endoscopy etc should form a part of periodic health examination.
5. Provision for after care and rehabilitation of cancer patients should also be kept in mind.

Treatment

Treatment of cancer depends on its type and stage:
1. Surgery is the most common approach for treatment of cancers, which are confined to one location and have not spread, for example skin cancers, lung cancer, breast cancer, cancer of colon.
2. Radiation and/or chemotherapy are used in combination with surgery when surgery alone cannot remove all of the cancer.
3. The cancer of lymph gland, lymphoma is treated most commonly with chemotherapy and radiation therapy while surgery is rarely used.

Cancer Control Program was undertaken in 1965 through six regional centers in the country:
1. Tata Memorial Cancer Hospital, Mumbai
2. Radiation Institute, Patna
3. Chittranjan National Cancer Research Center, Kolkata
4. M.P. Shah Cancer Hospital, Ahmedabad
5. Missionary Cancer Institute, Vellore
6. Barnanrd Institute of Radiology, Chennai.

DIABETES

Diabetes is a heterogeneous group of diseases characterized by hyperglycemia (high blood sugar concentration) and glucosuria (excretion of sugar in urine). It is due to deficiency or lack of insulin secretion or its ineffectiveness, which results in impaired metabolism of the nutrients, especially that of carbohydrates. Diabetes is essentially the disease of old and middle age, about 70–80% diabetes patients being above 50 years of age. The estimated prevalence in India is 1%.

Causes and risk factors

The causes and risk factors of diabetes are discussed below:

1. Etiology is not clear but certainly there is defective secretion of insulin and its utilization.
2. Insulin is a hormone that controls blood sugar and is secreted by pancreas. Insulin moves the glucose from blood stream into muscle, fat and liver cells where it serves as a source of energy for the body.
3. People suffering from diabetes have high blood sugar level due to insufficient or no secretion of insulin from pancreas or cells do not respond to insulin or both.
4. Diabetes mellitus is predominantly derangement of carbohydrates metabolism and to a lesser extent that of fat and proteins.
5. Diabetes is hereditary disorder.
6. Obesity is important in diabetes.
7. Diet rich in carbohydrates and fats aggravates diabetes.
8. Fast urbanization increasing stress and strain in life and sedentary habits contribute to increase in incident of diabetes. Death rate in diabetes increases with age.

Types of diabetes

There are three major types of diabetes:

Type of diabetes	Characteristics
Type 1 (*Insulin-dependent diabetes mellitus (IDDM) or Juvenile diabetes*)	1. In this type body makes little or no insulin. 2. Most often diagnosed in children, teens or young adults although can occur at any age. 3. Exact cause of this type is unknown. 4. Patients need daily injection of insulin.
Type 2 (*Non-insulin-dependent diabetes mellitus or Adult onset diabetes*)	1. In this type fat, liver and muscle cells do not respond correctly to insulin. 2. It is the most common form of diabetes. 3. Most often occurs in adulthood. 4. Therapy of *type 2* diabetes aims at first lowering high blood glucose level.

(Contd.)

Gestational *diabetes*	This type includes pregnant women who do not have diabetes but develop high blood sugar at any time. It may precede development of *type 2* diabetes.

Symptoms

Symptoms of diabetes occur as a result of high blood sugar level:

1. Blurred vision
2. Fatigue
3. Excessive thirst
4. Frequent urination
5. Weight loss
6. Hunger.

Diagnosis

High blood sugar may be determined by urine test. If blood sugar level is higher than 200 mg/dL, then one or more of the following tests must be done for the confirmation of diabetes:

1. Fasting blood glucose level

Sugar level	Condition
> 126 mg/dL	Diabetes
100–126 mg/dL	Impaired fasting glucose or pre-diabetes

   These levels are risk factor for *type 2* diabetes.

2. Hemoglobin A1c test (Glycosylated hemoglobin): This is a laboratory test that shows the average amount of sugar in blood over 3 months. An HbA1c of 6% or less is normal.

Condition	Level
Normal	< 5.7 %
Pre-diabetes	5.7– 6.4 %
Diabetes	Equal to or more than 6.5 %

3. Oral glucose tolerance test: If glucose level is higher than 200 mg/dL after 2 hours than diabetes is diagnosed.

Treatment

For the management of *type 1* diabetes following measures must be undertaken:

1. People who have just been diagnosed may need to stay in the hospital.
2. Everyone with *type 1* diabetes must take insulin every day.
3. People with *type 1* diabetes should eat at about the same times each day and try to eat the same kinds of foods.
4. Management of blood sugar level.
5. Foot care: check and care for feet every day.

6. Prevention of complications like heart attack and stroke.
7. Do not smoke.

Treatment of *type 2* diabetes include following measures:

1. The main treatment is exercise and diet.
2. If diet and exercise do not help to keep blood sugar at normal or near-normal levels than doctor may prescribe medication, which include one or more of the following drugs:
   (a) *Sulfonylureas:* Glimepiride, Glyburide and Tolazamide
   (b) *Alpha-glucosidase inhibitors:* Acarbose
   (c) *Biguanides:* Metformin
   (d) *Injectable medicines:* Exenatide, Mitiglinide, Pramlinide, Sitagliptin and Saxagliptin
   (e) *Meglitinides:* Repaglinide and Nateglinide
   (f) *Thiazolidinediones:* Rosiglitazone and Pioglitazone

   These drugs may be given with insulin, or insulin may be used alone.

Prevention and control

There is no way to prevent *type 1* diabetes but *type 2* diabetes may be prevented by keeping an ideal body weight and an active life-style. Following measures are recommended:

1. Marriage counseling to avoid marriage of persons with known family traits.
2. Prevention of obesity with emphasis on pre-diabetics keeping their weight about 10% less than optimum for their age and sex.
3. Early diagnosis through regular checkups, especially any persons with sedentary habits and family traits. Such screening tests include urine examination two hours after meals and blood sugar estimation two hours after 50 g of glucose orally.
4. For control of diabetes the important steps are – diet control, physical exercise, anti-diabetic drugs and personal hygiene including care of feet and skin.

BLINDNESS

Blindness can be defined as a state when vision becomes less than 3/60th of normal vision or when a person is unable to count fingers in daylight at a distance of 3 meters. It is estimated that there are 15 million blind people in the world and 3 million in India.

Causes of blindness

The main causes of blindness are:

1. Communicable diseases like inflammation, ophthalmias, trachoma, smallpox, venereal diseases. In India smallpox and trachoma account for 60% and 20% blindness cases, respectively. Poverty, illiteracy, poor nutrition, superstition, inadequate health services etc add to problem.

2. Non-communicable diseases: cataract, glaucoma, malnutrition (vitamin A deficiency), age related macular degeneration, diabetic retinopathy, congenital abnormalities like childhood cataract, optic atrophy, ill effects of faulty posture, glare, poor lighting and refractory errors.
3. Abnormalities and injuries.
4. Genetic defects such as albinism, Leber's congenital amaurosis, etc.
5. Poisoning caused by intake of certain chemicals like methanol.
6. Willful actions such as an act of vengeance, torture, etc.

Prevention and control

Diseases responsible for blindness should be prevented. Vitamin A deficiency can be corrected by recommended doses of concentrated vitamin A. Early diagnosis and treatment of diseases likely to lead to blindness is also useful. General public should be given health education in eye care. Long term measures are aimed at improving the quality of life and modifying or attacking the factors responsible for the persistence of eye health problems e.g. proper sanitation, adequate safe water supply, adequate intake of vitamin A rich foods, and high standard of personal hygiene.

The National Program for Control of Blindness was launched in 1976.

CARDIOVASCULAR DISEASES

Cardiovascular diseases are non-communicable and include a number of diseases of heart and blood vessels such as heart diseases, vascular lesions affecting CNS and disease of arteries, hypertension, atheroscleorosis, disease of veins etc. Broadly these are the diseases of modern age associated with civilization and are increasing with it. Developing countries are now warned to take appropriate measures to avoid the epidemic of non-communicable disease likely to come with socio-economic and health development.

Risk factors

Major risk factors in cardiovascular diseases include:

1. Cigarette use and other forms of smoking.
2. Alcohol abuse.
3. Failure or inability to obtain preventive health services e.g. for hypertension control.
4. Life-style changes e.g. dietary patterns, physical activity.
5. Environmental risk factors like occupational hazards, air and water pollution etc.
6. Stress factors.
7. Age and gender.

Epidemiology

Each disease has its own epidemiological characteristic. Congenital heart disease is associated with (a) viral infection like German measles, measles and mumps, (b) exposure to radiation or radiomimetic or cytotoxic drugs, antimetabolites and other drugs like thalidomide etc. Rheumatic carditis is considered as manifestation of type A streptococcal infection. Cardiovascular syphilis, toxic myocarditis owing to diphtheria and subacute bacterial endocarditis owing to *Streptococcus viridans* are other problems due to infection.

Types

1. Coronary heart disease.
2. Cardiomyopathy.
3. Cardiovascular disease.
4. Ischaemic heart disease.
5. Heart failure.
6. Hypertensive heart disease.
7. Inflammatory heart disease.
8. Valvular heart disease.
9. Myocardial infarction.

Diagnosis

The following biomarkers are used to diagnose the risk of cardiovascular disease:

1. Higher fibrinogen and PAI-1 (plasminogen activator inhibitor) blood concentrations.
2. Elevated homocysteine, or even upper half of normal.
3. Elevated blood levels of asymmetric dimethylarginine.
4. Inflammation as measured by C-reactive protein.
5. Elevated blood levels of brain natriuretic peptide (BNP).

Prevention and control

Following measures are recommended:

1. Avoid exposures to radiation, antimetabolites and cytotoxic drugs, viral infection and immunization by living viral vaccines during first trimester of pregnancy for prevention of congenital heart diseases.
2. A low-fat high-fiber diet including whole grains and plenty of fresh fruit and vegetables.
3. A diet high in vegetables and fruits.
4. Tobacco cessation and avoidance of second-hand smoke.
5. Limit alcohol consumption to the recommended daily limits.
6. Lower blood pressure, if elevated, through the use of antihypertensive medications.
7. Decrease body fat if overweight or obese.
8. Increase daily activity to 30 minutes of vigorous exercise per day at least five times per week.
9. Decrease emotional stress.
10. Consumption of 1–2 standard alcoholic drinks per day may reduce risk by 30%.
11. All streptococcal infections should be promptly treated by chemotherapy.

STROKE

The rapidly developing loss of brain functions due to disturbance in the blood supply to the brain is medically termed as stroke. Symptoms of stroke generally start suddenly and mostly last in seconds to minutes. It is a medical emergency and can cause permanent neurological damage. Previously it was called as cerebrovascular accident. In this disease the affected area of the brain is unable to function, which finally results in:

    (i) inability to move one or more limbs on one side of the body, or

   (ii) inability to understand or formulate speech, or

  (iii) inability to see one side of the visual field.

According to World Health Organization stroke is defined as "neurological deficit of cerebrovascular cause that persists beyond 24 hours or is interrupted by death within 24 hours". In this definition the time frame of 24 hours has been chosen arbitrarily.

Etiology of stroke

(a) Ischemia: Lack of blood flow caused by blockage such as thrombosis, arterial embolism.

(b) Hemorrhage: Leakage of blood.

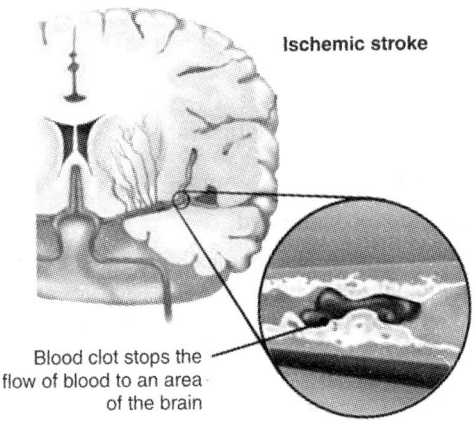

Ischemic stroke

Blood clot stops the flow of blood to an area of the brain

Fig. 8.1. Etiology of ischemic stroke.

Risk factors

1. Old age.
2. Hypertension (high blood pressure).
3. Previous stroke or transient ischemic attack.
4. Diabetes.
5. High cholesterol.
6. Cigarette smoking.
7. Atrial fibrillation.

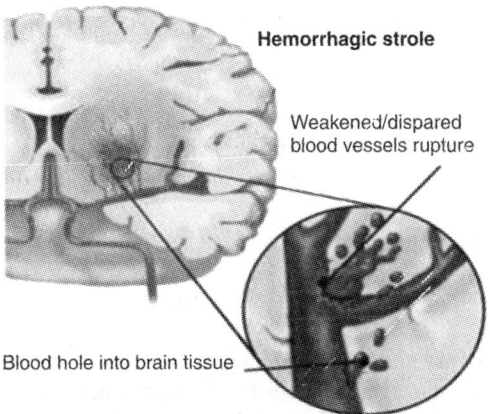

Fig. 8.2. Etiology of hemorrhagic stroke.

Classification of Strokes

Strokes can be classified into the following categories:

Ischemic stroke

These are the strokes, which are caused by interruption of the blood supply, leading to dysfunction of the brain tissue in that area. These are treated with thrombolysis. Reasons which might cause these strokes include:

1. Thrombosis.
2. Embolism.
3. Systemic hypo-perfusion.

Hemorrhagic stroke

These strokes result from rupture of a blood vessel or an abnormal vascular structure. Neurosurgery is the treatment of choice for hemorrhagic stroke. Hemorrhage is classified as:

1. Intracranial hemorrhage: accumulation of blood in the skull vault.
2. Intra-axial hemorrhage: accumulation of blood inside the brain.
3. Extra-axial hemorrhage: accumulation of blood inside the skull but outside the brain.

The main type of extra-axial hemorrhage are:

(a) Epidural hematoma: bleeding between the dura mater and the skull.
(b) Subdural hematoma: bleeding in the subdural space.
(c) Subarachnoid hemorrhage: bleeding between the arachnoid mater and pia mater.

Silent stroke

It is the stroke that does not have any outward symptoms. Although the patients are unaware of stroke but it still causes damage to the brain and patients are at increased risk factor for both transient ischemic attack and major stroke in future.

Diagnosis

Stroke is diagnosed by following techniques:

1. MRI scans.
2. CT scans.
3. Doppler ultrasound.
4. Arteriography.

Treatment

Patient having stroke should be admitted to "stroke unit", which is the ward of hospital staffed by nurses and therapists with experience in stroke management. Treatment depends on the reason which has caused the stroke i.e. ischemic or hemorrhagic.

Treatment strategies for ischemic stroke

Since the reason of ischemic stroke is occlusion of blood flow to artery supplying the brain leading to thrombus, hence therapy is directed to remove blockage by:

- *Thrombolysis*: Breaking down the clot known as thrombolysis. Tissue plasminogen activator (tPA) drugs are particularly used to dissolve the clot.
- *Thrombectomy*: Thrombectomy is the mechanical removal of thrombus. It is achieved by inserting a catheter into the femoral artery, directing it into cerebral circulation. Then a corkscrew-like device traps the clot and the clot is then removed from the body. This method has been found effective in patients not responding to or not able to take thrombolytic drugs.

    Anticoagulants are used to prevent recurrent stroke.

Treatment of hemorrhagic stroke

Neurosurgery is used to detect and treat the cause of hemorrhagic stroke. The treatment strategy (antithrombotics and anticoagulants) for ischemic stroke cannot be applied in hemorrhage, since they can make bleeding worse.

ASTHMA

It is the chronic inflammatory disease of airways characterized by reversible airflow obstruction and bronchospasm, due to tightening and swelling of muscles surrounding the airways. It is a disorder that causes airways of lungs to swell and narrow, leading to wheezing, shortness of breath, chest tightness and coughing.

Signs and symptoms

1. Wheezing.
2. Shortness of breath.

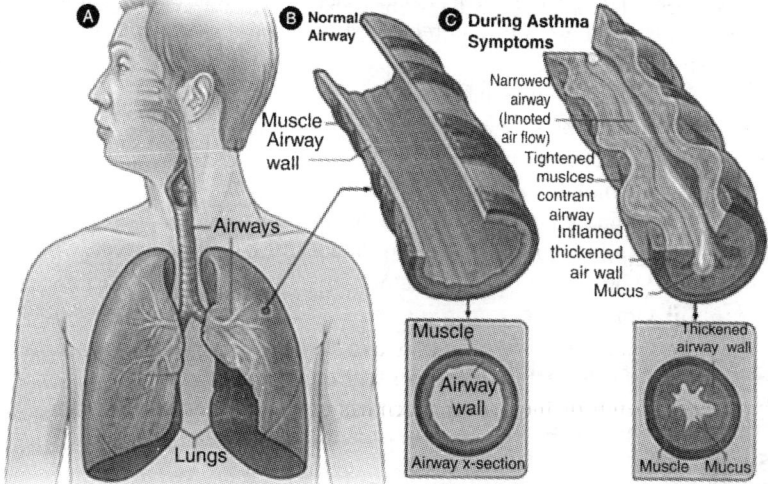

Fig. 8.3. Steps involved in provoking symptoms of asthma.

3. Chest tightness.
4. Cough.
5. Use of accessory muscle.
6. Bluish colour, extreme difficulty in breathing, rapid pulse, sweating and severe anxiety.

Risk factors

1. Allergens or triggers that cause allergy in sensitive people, for example dust, animals, changes in weather, chemicals, exercise, mold, pollen, respiratory infections, tobacco smoke, stress, etc.
2. Aspirin and other NSAIDs in some patients.
3. Personal or family history of allergies.

Tests for diagnosis

1. Arterial blood gas.
2. Chest X-ray.
3. Complete blood count.
4. Lung function tests.
5. Peak flow measurements.

Treatment

Treatment of asthma aims at following two strategies:

1. Avoidance of the allergens.
2. Control of airway inflammation: It includes two basic kinds of medication for treating asthma.

(a) Control drugs to prevent attacks. These drugs control the symptoms of asthma. These are required to be taken every day and include the following drugs:
  (i) Corticosteroids inhalers.
  (ii) Long-acting beta-agonist.
  (iii) Leukotriene inhibitors.
  (iv) Cromolyn sodium or Nedocromil sodium.
  (v) Aminophylline or Theophylline.
(b) Quick-relief drugs for use during attacks; also known as "rescue" drugs:
  (i) Short-acting bronchodilators.
  (ii) Oral steroids.

CHRONIC KIDNEY DISEASE

It is progressive loss of renal function over a period of months or years.

Symptoms

1. Feeling of unwell.
2. Reduced appetite.
3. High blood pressure.
4. Complications such as cardiovascular disease, anemia, pericarditis, diabetes.

Diagnosis

1. Blood test for creatinine.
2. Medical imaging.
3. Renal biopsy.
4. Abdominal ultrasound.
5. Nuclear medicine MAG3 (mercapto acetyl tri glycine) scan.
6. DMSA (technetium dimercaptosuccinic acid) scan.

Risk factors

1. Diabetes mellitus.
2. Hypertension.
3. Glomerulonephritis.

Classification of kidney diseases

1. Vascular: Renal artery stenosis, hemolytic-uremic syndrome, vasculitis.
2. Glomerular:
    (a) Primary glomerular disease: Focal segmental glomerulosclerosis, IgA nephritis.
    (b) Secondary glomerular disease: Diabetic nephropathy, lupus nephritis.
3. Tubulointerstitial: Polycystic kidney disease, drug and toxin-induced chronic tubulointerstitial nephritis, reflux nephropathy.
4. Obstructive disease: Bilateral kidney stones, disease of prostate.

Stages

There are three criteria for individuals suffering from chronic kidney disease.

1. Patients having glomerular filtration rate (GFR) of less than 60 mL/min/ 1.73 m^2 for 3 months are considered to have chronic kidney disease.
2. Individuals with kidney disease with any level of GFR are considered to be suffered from chronic kidney disease.
3. Loss of protein in the urine.

Stage	Characteristics
1	Kidney damage, slightly diminished function, normal or high GFR (> or = 90 mL/min/1.73 m^2)
2	Kidney damage, mild reduction in GFR (60–89 mL/min/1.73 m^2)
3	Moderate reduction in GFR (30–59 mL/min/1.73 m^2)
4	Severe reduction in GFR up to 15–29 mL/min/1.73 m^2
5	Kidney failure with GFR less than 15 mL/min/1.73 m^2

Treatment

Therapy of chronic kidney disease aims at:
    (i) to slow down the progression of disease, and
    (ii) treatment of original disease.

ALZHEIMER'S DISEASE

It is the form of dementia, which affects memory, thinking and behavior of patients and gets worse gradually with time. It is also known as *senile dementia of the Alzheimer type* or *primary dementia of the Alzheimer type.*

Symptoms

1. Memory impairment.
2. Language problems.
3. Inability in making decision.
4. Problems related to judgment and personality.

Risk factors

1. Age.
2. Family history (genetic factors).
3. Long-standing high blood pressure.
4. History of head trauma.
5. Environmental factors.
6. Female gender.

Types of Alzheimer's disease

Characteristics	Early onset Alzheimer's disease	Late onset Alzheimer's disease
1. Development of symptoms	Before age 60	At age of 60 and older
2. Incidence	Less common	More common than early onset Alzheimer's disease
3. Prognosis	It tends to progress rapidly	It progress comparatively slow
4. Cause	This disease can run in family, several genes have been found responsible	Disease may run in some families but role of gene is not very clear

Pathophysiology

In Alzheimer's disease neurons are destroyed, which results in decrease of neurotransmitters. These changes lead to the disconnection of areas of brain, which normally work together.

Following changes are commonly observed in the brain tissues of person died of Alzheimer's disease:

1. Neurofibrillary tangles.
2. Neuritic plaques.
3. Senile plaques.

Diagnosis

1. A skilled doctor or nurse can diagnose Alzheimer's disease through a history and physical examination based on presence of characteristic neurological and neuropsychological features and the absence of alternative conditions.
2. Thyroid disease, vitamin deficiency, brain tumor, stroke, intoxication from medication, chronic infection, anemia and severe depression are some other diseases, which can cause dementia. Test must be performed to determine that dementia is not caused by these diseases.
3. Dementia caused by other conditions like brain tumor or stroke may be determined by computed tomography (CT) or magnetic resonance imaging (MRI) and single photon emission tomography (SPECT) or positron emission tomography (PET).
4. In non-imaging biomarkers, decreased level of NAA/Cr and decreased hippocampal glutamate may be an early indication of Alzheimer's disease. (NAA = Glucose/N-acetylaspartate; Cr = Glucose/creatinine)

Treatment

Unfortunately, Alzheimer's disease is incurable and degenerative. So treatment of Alzheimer aims at:

1. Slowing the progression of disease.
2. Management of:
   - Behavior problems
   - Confusion
   - Sleep problems
   - Agitation
3. Friendly environment
4. Support of family and friends.

The first strategy, that is, slowing the progression of disease, is achieved by use of drugs, but benefit of these drugs is often small and even not noticeable. Drug should be used on the basis of benefit to risk ratio.

There are two categories of drugs, which are used in treatment of Alzheimer's disease:

1. Anticholinergic drugs: These drugs reduce the level of acetylcholine in the brain.
   - Drugs which come in this category are Donepezil, Rivastigmine, Galantamine.
   - Side effects of these drugs are: Indigestion, diarrhea, loss of appetite, nausea, vomiting, muscle cramps and fatigue.
2. Memantine: It is a novel class of drug, which is used in Alzheimer's disease. It acts on glutamatergic system by blocking NMDA glutamate receptors.
   - Side effects: Agitation or anxiety.

Prevention

Although there is no specific way to prevent Alzheimer's disease yet following measures may be followed in daily routine by a person belonging to a family with history of dementia:

1. Consumption of a low-fat diet.
2. Reduce consumption of linoleic acid.
3. Take food rich in omega-3 fatty acids.
4. Increased intake of darkly colored fruits and vegetables containing antioxidants such as carotenoids, vitamin E and vitamin C.
5. Involve actively and mentally in social life.

CHAPTER

9

Epidemiology

INTRODUCTION

Epidemiology is the basic science of prevention and social medicine evolved rapidly during the last 50 years. Epidemiology (*epi* – upon; *demon* – people) is defined as a study of any phenomenon among people and here we are concerned with the phenomenon of disease. According to WHO, *epidemiology is the study of the distribution and determinants of health-related states or events (including disease), and the application of this study to the control of diseases and other health problems.* Various methods can be used to carry out epidemiological investigations: surveillance and descriptive studies can be used to study distribution and analytical studies are used to study determinants. The main objectives of epidemiology are prevention, control and complete eradication of disease from the human race. Pharmacists are equally concerned with communicable and non-communicable disease.

Epidemiology is concerned with the detailed study of disease or other abnormalities in medical science, especially in respect of its agent, host, environment and distribution relationship. Epidemiology is also concerned with the measurement of health-related events and states in the community e.g. health needs, demands, activities, and variables such as blood pressure, serum cholesterol, height, weight etc. The ultimate aim of epidemiology is twofold:

1. To eliminate or reduce the health problem or its consequence.
2. To promote the health and well being of society as a whole.

Three **basic components** of epidemiology are:

1. Study of disease frequency.
2. Study of the distribution of disease.
3. Study of determinant of the disease.

Epidemiology involves the following **steps:**

1. Design of studies.
2. Collection and statistical analysis of data.
3. Interpretation and dissemination of results.

Epidemiology includes the following **areas** in the study of disease:

1. Outbreak investigation.
2. Disease surveillance and screening of medicine.
3. Biomonitoring.
4. Comparison of treatment effects.
5. Biology of disease process.
6. Biostatistics.
7. Exposure assessment.
8. Social science.

Epidemiology covers the description and causation of disease in general (not only epidemic disease) including non-disease health-related conditions, for example, high blood pressure and obesity.

METHODS OF EPIDEMIOLOGY

The methods used in epidemiology are:

(a) Descriptive
(b) Analytical
(c) Experimental.

Descriptive and analytical epidemiology are also classified as observation studies.

A. Descriptive Epidemiology

It is the study and distribution of a disease i.e. time, place and people affected (when, where and who).

Procedures in descriptive epidemiology

1. Defining the population to be studied.
2. Defining the disease under study.
3. Describing the disease by time (seasonal, yearly, over few years, over a long period), place (topographical situation), person (age, sex, socio-economic profiles, occupation, etc).
4. Measurement of disease.
5. Comparison with known indices.
6. Formation of etiological hypothesis.

Once an etiological hypothesis is formulated, the actual factors and modes of transmission of a disease are easily arrived at. Descriptive epidemiology provides data for planning, organizing and evaluating prevention and curative services.

B. Analytical Epidemiology

It is concerned with the study of a disease in respect of its source of origin, route of transmission and its extent of spread (what, how and how much). The study comprises of three distinctive types of observation studies:

(a) Case series study.
(b) Case control study.
(c) Cohort study.

(a) Case series study

Case series study is the qualitative study of the experience of a single patient, or small group of patients with a similar diagnosis, or to a statistical technique comparing periods during which patients are exposed to some factor with the potential to produce illness with periods when they are unexposed. From these studies a clinician identifies an unusual feature of a disease or a patient's history leading to formulation of a new hypothesis while the former type of studies were purely descriptive and cannot be used to make inferences about the general population of patients with that disease.

(b) Case control study

Case control studies are also called *retrospective* studies. These are backward studies which are usually made out of records. The focus is on a disease or some other health problem that has already developed. Case control studies involve cases and controls and the unit is the individual rather than the group. Before the start of the study both exposure and outcome (disease) have already occurred and the study proceeded backward from effect to cause. Cases and controls must be comparable with respect to known factors such as age, sex, social status etc. In the first step a suitable group of cases and a group controls are identified. In the second step selected cases and control are matched with respect to particular factors.

(c) Cohort study

Cohort means a group of people having a common characteristic or experience within a definite time period. Thus people born in 2010 form birth cohort of 2010, people married in 2010 form marriage cohort of 2010, and those exposed to a particular infection in 2010 form exposure cohort of 2010. Cohort study is also known as *prospective* study, longitudinal study or forward looking study. Such studies are made with a view to highlight risk factors through a comparison of control and experimental groups.

C. Experimental Epidemiology

It involves experimental studies in laboratory animals or human population. Experimental studies are conducted in a scientific way using statistical designs. Evaluation of polio vaccine in a group of population is an experimental prospective study aimed at evaluating role of polio vaccine through comparison with a control population group without the vaccine.

USES OF EPIDEMIOLOGY

Techniques of epidemiology have application in the areas of disease, health and health services. Important uses of epidemiology are:

1. It provides a means to study disease profiles and trends in human population. This is useful in identifying emerging health problems based on historical study of the rise and fall of disease in the population. It enables to forecast the future trends of disease and their prevalence, for example increasing incidence of malaria during rainy season and cyclic incidence of small pox.

2. It is a diagnostic tool of community medicine and is useful in community diagnosis. The term community diagnosis refers to the identification and quantitation of health problems in a community. It also brings forward the relation of various diseases to certain factors like relation of smoking to cancer.

3. It makes possible to know the types of diseases prevalent in a community. The time, place, seasonal incidence and environment factors can also be noted. The extent of morbidity and mortality caused by the disease is known.

4. It is useful in planning and evaluation of health services. Planning includes planning facilities for medical care, for example number of hospital beds required for patients with specific disease, planning facilities for preventive services e.g. immunization campaigns etc. The effectiveness of any measures to control or prevent a disease is determined by evaluation.

5. Epidemiology is useful in assessing individuals' risk and chance in a population, for example risk assessment for smokers as a cause of death by cancer.

6. Epidemiological investigations are useful in defining and identification of syndromes. Differentiation of gastric and duodenal ulcers has been possible by epidemiological studies. Similarly misconception about any disease syndrome can be removed by epidemiology.

7. Epidemiology gives the complete picture of disease in a population. It studies the disease pattern in the community in relation to agent, host and environment factors and hence gives a better picture of the natural history of disease. This is particularly important in chronic disease like ischemic heart disease where most of the deaths are sudden. As most of the patients are unable to reach the hospital, a clinician doesn't get the complete information. Epidemiological perspective of a disease is broadest.

8. Epidemiological studies identify the causes of disease and risk factors by relating disease to inter-population difference and other attributes of the population.

9. It forms the basis to set up various physiological and anatomical standards, for example, in respect of height and weight of various ages, blood pressure etc.

10. Epidemiological study offers a scope of research facilities for experimental studies in the field of medical sciences.

DYNAMICS OF DISEASE TRANSMISSION

A communicable disease is one in which the causative organism may pass or be carried from one person to another or from one animal to another, either directly or indirectly. Communicable diseases are transmitted from source (reservoir) of infection to the susceptible host by different modes of transmission. Passing of a communicable disease from an infected host, individual or group, to a nonspecific individual or group, is known as transmission. Study of disease transmission is essential for implementing proper infection control measures. The relationship is represented in Fig. 9.1.

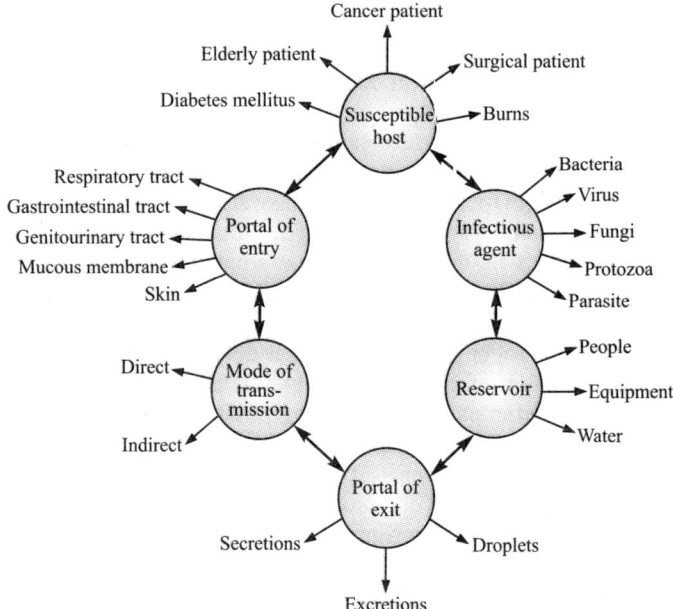

Fig. 9.1. Chain of infection.

A. RESERVOIRS OF INFECTION

(a) Source and reservoir

The **source** of infection may be a person, animal, object or substance from which an infective agent passes to the host. **Reservoir** is the natural habitat of the infective organism. It may be a person, animal, arthropod, plant, soil or substance in which the infective agent lives and multiplies. The reservoir may be three types – *human, animal* and *non-living things*. The term source refers to the immediate source of infection, which may or may not be part of reservoir. In tetanus the source and reservoir are the same i.e. soil. In hookworm infection source of infection is the soil contaminated with infective larvae but reservoir is man.

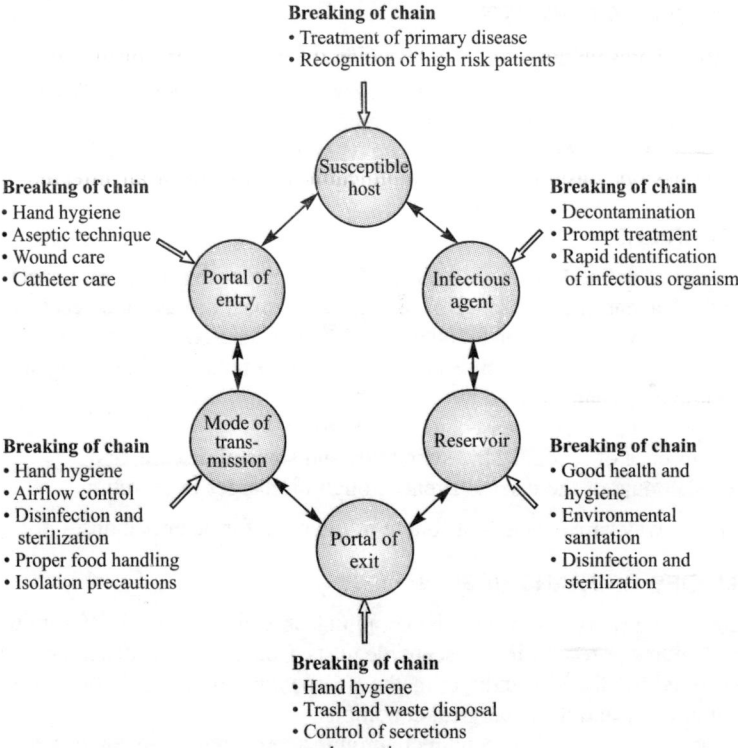

Fig. 9.2. Breaking of chain of infection to prevent infection.

(i) Human reservoirs

Many people carry pathogens and transmit them to others, directly or indirectly. These people may have signs and symptoms of the disease; or they may be in a period without signs and symptoms, either before or after the disease develops. Others may be carriers without ever developing signs or symptoms of the disease, which are known as *asymptomatic carriers*.

(ii) Animal reservoirs

Zoonoses are diseases which are primarily diseases of animals, but can be transmitted to humans. About 15 zoonoses have been identified, and these diseases spread to humans in various ways:

(a) Direct contact with infected animals.
(b) Direct contact with waste of pets (for example, cleaning kitty box).
(c) Contamination of food or water.
(d) Contact with contaminated hides, feathers, or fur.
(e) By consuming infected animal products.
(f) By insect vectors.

(iii) Non-living reservoirs

The two main examples are soil and water.

1. Soil: Fungus organisms (ringworm and systemic infections); *Clostridium botulinum, Clostridium tetani* are common.
2. Water: *Vibrio cholerae, Salmonella typhi*, other gastrointestinal diseases – usually the water gets contaminated by feces of humans or animals.

B. CARRIERS

A carrier is defined as an infected person or animal that harbors a specific infectious agent in the absence of discernible clinical disease and serves as a potential source of infection for others. This carrier state exists due to inadequate treatment or immune response and incomplete removal of disease agent. A carrier state is characterized by:

(a) presence of the disease agent in the body,
(b) absence of recognizable symptoms and signs of disease, and
(c) shedding of the disease agent through discharges or secretion.

In this way carrier acts as a source of infection for other persons.

C. MODES OF TRANSMISSION

There are many ways in which the communicable disease may be transmitted from a source or reservoir to susceptible hosts. Communicable disease may be transmitted by direct or indirect methods depending on the infectious agent, portal of entry and the ecological conditions.

Transmission can also be indirect, through another organism, either a vector (for example a mosquito) or an intermediate host (for example tapeworm in pigs can be transmitted to humans who ingest improperly cooked pork). Indirect transmission could involve zoonoses or, more typically, larger pathogens like macroparasites with more complex life cycles.

Classification

Transmission of disease is classified on the basis of mode of infection in the following classes:

(a) Contact transmission

Spread of an agent of disease by direct contact, indirect contact, or droplet. It includes direct touch (host to host or object to host) or exposure to a source of an infection, or a person who is exposed.

1. Direct transmission

The immediate transfer of an agent from a reservoir to a susceptible host by direct contact or droplet spread. In this type, transmission takes place from person-to-person without involvement of intermediate object, for example respiratory diseases, staphylococcal infections, hepatitis A, measles, smallpox, STDs including AIDS. Rabies and anthrax spread from animals to people.

(a) **Direct contact:** In this case the contact is direct between the source to the susceptible host without any intermediate agency. Direct contact is established through touching, kissing, sexual intercourse etc. Thus shaking hands with an infected person can directly transmit the disease and hence the Indian system of greeting with *Namaskar* avoids transmission of infection. Examples of diseases transmitted by direct contact include AIDS, sexually transmitted disease (STD), skin and eye infection, and leprosy etc.

(b) **Droplet infection:** It is the direct transmission of an infectious agent from a reservoir to a susceptible host by spray with relatively large aerosols produced by sneezing, coughing, laughing or talking less than 1 meter. Droplets of saliva and nasopharyngeal secretion during sneezing, coughing or speaking and spitting are responsible for transmission of many diseases. Every cough or sneeze results into a microbe laden spray containing millions of bacteria and virus. The smallest spray droplets remain suspended for some time in the air and may be carried many feet by drafts. Diseases transmitted in this way include respiratory infection, enteric fever, many infections of the nervous system, whooping cough, common cold, diphtheria, influenza, pneumonia, tuberculosis, meningococcal meningitis etc.

(c) **Contact with soil:** Disease agent may be present in soil, compost or decaying vegetable matter and may be acquired by susceptible host on exposure. Spray droplets containing disease agent would ultimately settle down. Thus all the disease transmitted through droplets infection can also be transmitted through contact with soil.

2. Indirect transmission

Infection may be transmitted indirectly through the agency of a third person, through a vector or a vehicle. This includes the 5 F's: *f*lies, *f*ingers, *f*omites, *f*ood and *f*luid'. The infectious agent may be capable of surviving in the external environment till it finds a new host and must retain its pathogenicity and virulence till such time. Indirect transmission may be in-animate (contaminated objects like dishes, utensils, toys, books etc) or animate (insects, which are capable of carrying infection from one host to another such as plague, malaria, etc).

(a) **In-animate:**

　(i) *Fomites-borne:* Fomites are inanimate objects other than food or water, for example drinking glasses, door handles, lavatory chains, syringes, instruments, surgical dressings, soiled clothes, towels, linen, hand-kerchief, spoons, dishes, pencils, book etc. These objects get contaminated by the infectious discharges from a patient and transmit the infection to healthy users. Thus fomites can transmit bacillary dysentery, typhoid fever, diphtheria, hepatitis B, eye and skin infection.

　(ii) *Vehicle-borne:* Water, food, ice, blood, serum, plasma etc act as vehicles in the transmission of infection. Water and food are the most potential vehicles because they are used by everyone. Diseases transmitted by water and food include food poisoning, acute diarrhoea, typhoid fever, cholera, polio and hepatitis A, whereas hepatitis B, malaria, syphilis may be transmitted by blood. Organ transplantation may transmit cytomeogalovirus.

- Water-borne transmission: Pathogens usually originate in untreated or poorly treated sewage, for example cholera, shigellosis, leptospirosis.

- Food-borne transmission: Transmission in foods that are incompletely cooked, poorly refrigerated, and contaminated in preparation, for example food poisoning and tapeworm infestations.

(iii) *Air-borne:* It occurs when bacteria, viruses or other pathogens travel on dust particles or on small respiratory droplets that may become aerosolized when people sneeze, cough, laugh, or exhale. They hang in the air much like invisible smoke. Air borne infection may be transmitted through droplet nuclei and dust. *Droplets nuclei* are tiny particles (1 to 10 µm) representing the dried droplets during sneezing, coughing etc. Being so tiny in size, droplet nuclei remain suspended in air for long time and may be carried over distances through air currents. In airborne transmission spread of agents takes place by droplets that travel more than 1 meter from the reservoir to the new host. Droplets nuclei in the size range of 1 to 5 µm may enter into the alveoli of the lungs. Tuberculosis, influenza, chickenpox, measles, Q fever and many respiratory infections are transmitted in this manner. Large droplets settle down on the objects in the environment and become part of the dust. Many infectious agents like streptococci, staphylococci, pathogenic bacteria, virus and fungal spores can survive in the dust for considerable periods. This contaminated dust is swirled during sweeping, dusting etc and the dust comes into the air. Streptococcal and staphylococcal infections, pneumonia, tuberculosis, Q fever and psittacosis, many fungal diseases etc may be transmitted through dust and this is very important in hospital infections.

(iv) *Hands and fingers:* Unclean hands and fingers show lack of personal hygiene. Milkers, dairyman and cooks can act as carrier of respiratory or intestinal infectious microorganism by infecting milk supplies and food. Shaking unclean hands may transmit many pathogenic organisms like poliomyelitis, bacillary dysentery and respiratory disease. Hands must be washed after defecation, urination or blowing the nose.

(b) **Animate:** *Vector-borne:* Vectors are animal or any living carrier that transmit pathogens from one host to another or an animate intermediate host in the indirect transmission of an agent that carries the agent from a reservoir to a susceptible host. Often they are arthropods (insects, ticks, mites). A few examples of diseases transmitted by vectors are malaria, yellow fever, Lyme disease, and Rocky Mountain spotted fever.

Vector-borne transmission may be of two types:

1. Mechanical transmission: Pick up the pathogen and carry it on feet or other body parts, for example, flies.
2. Biological transmission: Pathogen must undergo a necessary stage of development inside the body of the vector, for example, mosquitoes.

Transmission of vector-borne infection may involve following **chains**.

- Man – arthropod – man (malaria)
- Man – snail – man (schistosomiasis)
- Mammal – arthropod – man (plague)
- Bird – arthropod – man (encephalitis)
- Man – cyclops – fish – man (fish tapeworm)
- Man – snail – fish – man (clonorchis simenesis)
- Man – snail – crab – man (paragonimiasis)

Vector may also transmit infectious agent by biting, regurgitation, scratching-in of infective faces and contamination of host with their body fluids. Arthropods that fly or crawl may mechanically transmit intestinal and other disease organisms on their feet and bodies.

D. VERTICAL TRANSMISSION

Transmission of disease from an infected mother to the fetus either during pregnancy, childbirth *via* the placenta, or by breast-feeding is known as vertical transmission, which include rubella virus, herpes virus, syphilis and hepatitis B.

E. HORIZONTAL TRANSMISSION

Transmission of an infection from one person to another of the same generation in the same population.

F. CHANNELS OF INFECTION

Routes of entry of infection in the body are called channels of infection. The infection enters through three channels:

1. Through skin, for example, tetanus, rabies, syphilis, gonorrhea, malaria, plague, dengue, filariasis.
2. By inhalation, for example, diphtheria, whooping cough, measles, influenza, common cold, pulmonary tuberculosis, etc.
3. By ingestion, for example, diarrhea, dysentery, cholera, enteric fever.

PRINCIPLES OF DISEASE CONTROL AND PREVENTION

As we have seen earlier, there are three essential components in the chain of infection (Fig. 9.1):

1. Source or reservoir
2. Mode of transmission
3. Susceptible host.

Direct control and prevention is based on attacking any component and breaking the chain (Fig. 9.2). A single method or a combination of methods can be employed.

Disease control involves all the measures designed to prevent or reduce the incident, prevalence and consequence of disease. Complete knowledge about the etiology of a disease facilitates its control and prevention.

A. Controlling the Reservoir

The simplest method of controlling a disease would be elimination of a reservoir or source whenever possible. General measures of reservoir control in humans include early diagnosis, notification, isolation, treatment, quarantine, surveillance or disinfection.

1. Early diagnosis

Rapid identification is the first step in the control of communicable diseases. Diagnosis may be confirmed by laboratory tests. Early diagnosis is essential for the treatment of the patients for epidemiological investigation to study the time, place and person distribution and for the prevention and control measures.

2. Notification

Detection or even suspicion of a disease must be followed by notification by local health authority. The list of notifiable diseases usually includes those which are considered to cause serious harm to public health. It is an important source of epidemiological information. Notification helps in early detection of disease outbreaks and allows health authority to take immediate action to control their spread.

3. Epidemiological investigation

Epidemiology is the science that studies when and where diseases occur and how they are transmitted. This science began when Dr. John Snow traced an outbreak of cholera to contaminated water in London in 1848–1849. Epidemiology is concerned with the identification of the source of infection and factors, which influence its spread in the community e.g. geographical situation; climatic condition, social, cultural and behavioral patterns, the character of the disease agent; reservoir, the vectors and vehicles, and the susceptible host populations. An epidemiologist looks for the cause of the disease, the original source, and the connection between cases of the disease, as well as any other factors that might help in understanding of a disease outbreak. The next step is ending a current outbreak and preventing outbreaks in the future.

4. Isolation

Isolation is defined as separation for the period of communicability of infected persons or animals from others in such places and under such conditions as to prevent or limit the direct or indirect transmission of the infectious agent from those infected to those who are susceptible or who may spread the agent to others. Isolation prevents the transfer of infection from the reservoir to the possible susceptible hosts and thus protects the community. The duration of isolation is determined by the duration of communicability of the disease and the effect of chemotherapy on infectivity. Recommended periods of isolation for some common disease are given in Table 9.3.

Table 9.3. Recommended periods of isolation

Disease	Duration of isolation
Cholera	3 days after tetracycline started
Chickenpox	Until lesions crusted; usually about 6 days after the onset of rash
Diphtheria	Until 48 hours after antibiotics (or negative cultures after treatment)
Hepatitis A	3 weeks
Influenza	3 days after onset
Measles	From the onset of catarrhal through third day of rash
Mumps	Until sweating subsides
Polio	Children – 6 weeks, adults – 2 weeks
Tuberculosis (sputum +)	Until 3 weeks of effective chemotherapy

Although isolation is the oldest method of disease control, it is recommended only when the risk of transfer of the infection is exceptionally serious.

5. Treatment

It is aimed at killing the infectious agent before it is disseminated i.e. when it is still in the reservoir. It reduces the communicability of the disease, cuts short the duration of illness and prevents development of secondary care. Treatment is also extended to carriers. Treatment could be rendered to the individuals (individual treatment) or to all the persons in the community (mass treatment).

6. Quarantine

It is defined as the limitation of freedom of movement of such well persons or domestic animals exposed to communicable disease for a period of time, not longer than the longest usual incubation period of disease in such manner as to prevent effective contact with those not so exposed. It applies to restriction on the healthy contacts of an infectious disease. It is an outdated method of disease control.

B. Interruption of Transmission

This means preventing the infectious agent from a patient or carrier from entering the body of susceptible person by changing some component of human environment. Thus the chain of transmission is broken. For example, treatment of polluted water can interrupt transmission of many diseases like typhoid, dysentery, cholera, gastroenteritis, hepatitis A. Transmission of food-borne disease can be prevented by adequate cooking, promoting refrigeration of cooked foods and withdrawal of contaminated foods. In case of vector-borne diseases control measures should be directed primarily at the vector and its breeding places. Vector control includes destruction of stray dogs, control of cattle, pets and other animals so that spread of infection through them could be minimized. Thus blocking the routes of transmission implies an attack on environmental factors.

C. The Susceptible Host

The susceptible host or people at risk can be protected by:

1. Active immunization
2. Passive immunization
3. Combined active and passive immunization, for example simultaneous administration of hepatitis B vaccine and hepatitis B immunoglobulin
4. Chemoprophylaxis
5. Non-specific measures.

Prophylaxis means protection from or prevention of disease. *Chemoprophylaxis* means prophylaxis (protection) from infection through the use of drugs (chemical substances). *Causal prophylaxis* means complete prevention of infection by early elimination of causal agent. There is no causal prophylaxis against malaria. *Clinical prophylaxis* is the prevention of clinical symptoms and does not necessarily mean elimination of infection.

Non-specific measures include improvement in the quality of life such as better housing, water supply, sanitation, nutrition, education etc. Such measures have been largely responsible in the decline of tuberculosis, cholera, leprosy and child mortality. Community involvement is yet another important non-specific measure calling for the involvement of community in disease surveillance, disease control and public health activities. Over and above these measures, there is need to bring about changes in human behavior to disease control and life styles of the people. These are, in fact, major obstacles in disease control but can be overcome by educating the public.

Strategies for controlling a disease

These include:

1. Use of drugs
2. Immunization
3. Control of reservoirs of infection
4. Water treatment
5. Sewage disposal
6. Cold storage of food
7. Adequate cooking
8. Food inspection
9. Pasteurization

Portals of Exit

Microbes have preferred portals of entry and exit from the body of a host. Following are the measure portals of exit for microbes:

1. Respiratory tract: Pathogens living in this area are carried out by a cough or a sneeze. The list includes tuberculosis, whooping cough, pneumonia, smallpox, and influenza.
2. Gastrointestinal tract:
   (a) *Feces:* Salmonellosis, cholera, typhoid fever, shigellosis, polio, amoebic dysentery;
   (b) *Saliva:* Rabies.
3. Urogenital tract:
   (a) STDs in secretions from penis and vagina;
   (b) Typhoid fever and brucellosis in urine.
4. Drainage from wounds
5. Infected blood

IMMUNE SYSTEM

The body has its own complex system of cells, tissues and organs, which work together to protect itself against the attack of foreign invaders such as microbes like bacteria, parasites and fungi that can cause infections. This system is known as immune system. The organs of the immune systems are known as lymphoid organs since they are residence of key cells of immune system i.e. lymphocytes.

Self and Non-self

Success of immune system lies in its ability to distinguish between body's own cells, recognized as *self*, and foreign cells as *non-self*. The body's immune defenses normally coexist peacefully with cells that carry distinctive self marker molecules. But when immune defenders encounter foreign cells or organisms carrying markers that say 'non-self', they quickly launch an attack.

IMMUNITY

A large number and variety of microorganism are present in the environment and even in the body cavities. Infection occurs when microorganisms successfully invade the body and cause damage to the tissue.

Immunity

The ability of the body to resist and overcome infection is called immunity and the study of immunity is called *immunology*. Immunity is defined as the ability of the body to recognize, destroy and eliminate antigenic material, foreign to its own. When a person is immune to a specific infectious agent he does not suffer from that disease when the agent invades his body i.e. he is protected against that disease.

Antigen

An antigen is a foreign substance, which when introduced into the tissue, stimulates the production of a specific antibody and combines specifically with the antibody so formed. Antigen is anything that can trigger the immune response including a microbe such as a virus, or a part of a microbe such as a molecule, tissues or cells from another person which carries non-self markers.

Antibody

Antibody is a molecule (also called an *immunoglobulin*) produced by a mature B cell (plasma cell) in response to an antigen. When an antibody attaches to an antigen, it helps the body to destroy or inactivate the antigen.

Antibodies are formed in response to the antigens in the body as a defense mechanism which is in addition to phagocytosis. Antibodies are specific in nature. They react with antigens in the body by various mechanisms and neutralize them.

An antibody is made up of two heavy chains and two light chains as shown in Fig. 9.3. The variable region, which differs from one antibody to the next, allows an antibody to recognize its matching antigen. Various **types of immunity** are given in Fig. 9.4.

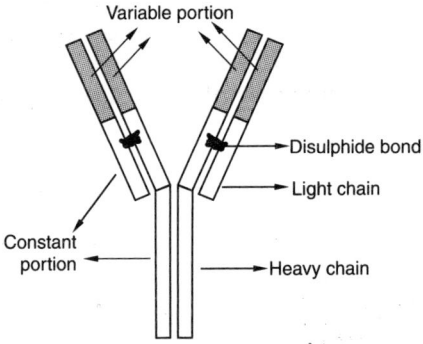

Fig. 9.3. Diagrammatic representation of an antibody.

Essentially antibodies are immunoglobulins and comprise the following five classes:

1. *Immunoglobulin G (IgG):* Antibody that works efficiently to coat microbes, speeding their uptake by other cells in the immune system.
2. *Immunoglobulin M (IgM):* Very effective at killing bacteria.
3. *Immunoglobulin A (IgA):* Concentrates in body fluids such as tears, saliva, and the secretions of the respiratory and digestive tracts, which guard the entrances to the body.
4. *Immunoglobulin E (IgE):* Mainly they protect against parasitic infections and are responsible for the symptoms of allergy.
5. *Immunoglobulin D (IgD):* Remain attached to B cells and play a key role in initiating early B cell responses.

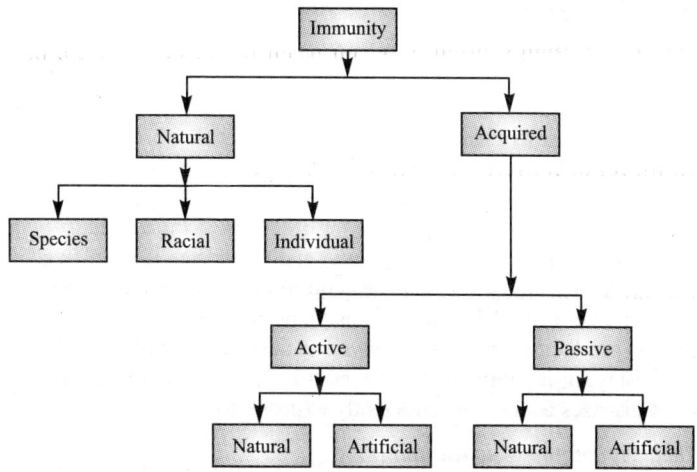

Fig. 9.4. Types of immunity.

A. Natural Immunity

It is the resistance to disease due to inherent constitutional make-up of an individual. It is not acquired due to the use of biologics. Levels of natural resistance to certain infectious diseases vary considerably among species, races and even among individuals as to age and sex.

1. *Species:* This type of natural resistance varies in species. However some disease like tuberculosis, anthrax, psittacosis and rabies etc occur both in animals and man alike. Man is susceptible to plague but fowls are not. Mice are not affected by typhoid fever but it is a serious disease in human beings. These differences in natural immunity are attributed to difference in species.

2. *Race:* Certain races of man are more susceptible to tuberculosis than other. Negros possess high resistance to yellow fever than white men. Negroes or white Indian are more susceptible to tuberculosis than Caucasian race.

3. *Individual:* Some people are more resistant to colds and skin infection than others. Most of the children in the age group of 2 to 5 years are susceptible to diphtheria but most adults are immune to it.

B. Acquired Immunity

Acquired immunity is developed in response to a specific stimulus. This immunity is needed because the natural immunity is inadequate for protection against many microbial diseases. Such immunity is developed due to the introduction of foreign substance or the immune substance produced in other individuals or in another species. Thus acquired immunity may be actively acquired due to the individuals antibody producing cells or passively acquired e.g. when the antibodies from another person or animals are introduced.

1. Active immunity

It may be either actively or passively acquired.

(a) Naturally acquired active immunity

It is acquired as a result of natural infection by pathogens either in a recognizable clinical presentation or a subclinical non-recognizable form. It is also acquired when a person recovers from certain disease e.g. after suffering from diphtheria, small pox or poliomyelitis, and persists for life whereas the immunity acquired after suffering from influenza, pneumonia and gonorrhea is short lived.

This type of immunity may also be acquired after subclinical infection due to smaller number of invading organisms. A person becomes immune because his antibody producing cells have received an adequate stimulus. Thus children and adults staying in slums develop naturally acquired active immunity to a variety of diseases as they are frequently exposed to sub-infections.

(b) Artificially acquired active immunity

This type of immunity is acquired by administration of antigens, usually by injection. The antigens used in this way are known as *vaccines* and may be microorganisms or their products. Administration of antigens stimulates formation of antibodies and immunity is acquired.

2. Passive immunity

Passive immunity may also be acquired either naturally or artificially.

(a) Naturally acquired passive immunity

Antibodies formed in a mother in response to a disease may be transferred to the fetus through the placental blood. This provides immunity to the infant for several months. This also explains why the babies are highly resistant for about six months to diphtheria, measles, chickenpox and scarlet fever.

(b) Artificially acquired passive immunity

This type of immunity is acquired by injecting the biological preparations known as antisera, sera or immune sera. These products are the antibodies produced in an animal, usually a horse, and occasionally in human beings. Passive immunity is not long lasting.

IMMUNIZATION

Immunization is the process of conferring immunity. It comprises of administering antigens for the purpose of stimulating a protecting antibody response. Vaccination is a form of immunization. Immunization is responsible for complete eradication of small pox and polio in India. Immunization program can be successful with the cooperation of government, voluntary agencies (for example NGOs; Non Government Organizations) and medical profession. Every Primary Health Centre (PHC) should have immunization facilities. In 1978 Government of India started the Expanded Program on Immunization

(EPI) covering six diseases – diphtheria, whooping cough, tetanus, polio, tuberculosis and measles. Small pox and polio have already been completely eradicated from India through such immunization program. The agents or products through which immunization is achieved are called *immunizing agents*. The immunizing agents or immunological products are classified as vaccines, immunoglobulins and sera.

Vaccination is used by healthcare providers to help the body's immune system prepare for future attacks. Vaccines could be either live attenuated vaccines or inactivated or killed vaccines prepared from bacteria, viruses or rickettsiae. Vaccines are also prepared from endotoxins produced by certain organisms (e.g. diphtheria and tetanus) by detoxifying these toxins. Vaccination remains one of the best ways to prevent infectious diseases, and vaccines have an excellent safety record. Previously devastating diseases such as smallpox, polio, and whooping cough have been greatly controlled or eliminated through worldwide vaccination programs. All antibodies are immunoglobulins and hence immunoglobulin preparations are also used for passive immunization. Antisera or immune sera are the preparations, which contain antibodies. These preparations are made in animals like horse (for a detailed account of immunological products please refer Text book of Professional Pharmacy by Jain and Sharma, Vallabh Prakasan, Delhi).

Expanded Program on Immunization to protect all children of the world was launched in India in January 1978. The program is now called Universal Child Immunization Program, 1990. The National Immunization Schedule is given in Table 9.1 and the WHO Immunization Schedule is given in Table 9.2.

Disorders of Immune System

These are:

(a) Allergic diseases
(b) Autoimmune diseases
(c) Immune complex diseases
(d) Immune deficiency diseases.

Immune deficiency diseases have been discussed below.

(a) Allergic diseases

Allergic diseases are the result of response of immune system to a false alarm. Allergic reactions are mediated by the antibodies belonging to class IgE. In allergic diseases, usually harmless substances are mistaken as threat and attacked by the immune system. The general examples of such allergic substances include house dust, grass pollen, food particles and mold etc.

(b) Autoimmune diseases

In autoimmune diseases the recognition apparatus of immune system is upset and hence body starts the production of T cells and antibodies against its own cells and tissues. These T cells and antibodies are known as misguided T cells

Table 9.1. National Immunization Schedule

Beneficiaries	Age	Vaccine	No. of doses	Route of administration
Infants	6 weeks to 9 months	DPT	3	Intramuscular
		Polio	3	Oral
		BCG	1$^\#$	Intradermal
	9 to 12 months	Measles		Subcutaneous
Children	16 to 24 months	DPT	1$^{\#\#}$	Intramuscular
		Polio	1$^{\#\#}$	Oral
	5 to 6 years	DT	1*	Intramuscular
		Typhoid	2	Subcutaneous
	10 years	Tetanus toxoid	1*	Intramuscular
		Typhoid	1*	Subcutaneous
	16 years	Tetanus toxoid	1*	Subcutaneous
		Typhoid	1*	Subcutaneous
Pregnant women	16 to 36 weeks	Tetanus toxoid	1*	Intramuscular

\# In case of institutional deliveries BCG to be given at birth
\#\# Booster dose
* Two doses, if not vaccinated previously

Note: Interval between 2 doses should not be less than 1 month. Minor coughs, colds and mild fever are not contraindications to vaccination.
Abbreviations: BCG = Bacillus Calmette Guerin; DPT = Diphtheria, Pertussis and Tetanus; DT = Diphtheria and Tetanus vaccine.

Table 9.2. WHO EPI Immunization Schedule*

Age	Vaccine
Birth	BCG, Oral polio
6 weeks 10 weeks 14 weeks	DPT, Oral polio
9 months	Measles

* When early protection is a must.

and autoantibodies, respectively and contribute many autoimmune disorders, for example rheumatoid arthritis, systemic lupus erythematosus (SLE), diabetes.

The exact causes of these diseases are not known but following factors are likely to be involved:

1. Environmental factors that may alter or damage normal body cells, for example viruses, sunlight and certain drugs.

2. Hormones.
3. Heredity, etc.

(c) Immune complex diseases

The clusters of interlocking antigens and antibodies are known as immune complex. Generally, these immune complexes are readily removed from blood circulation, but in some instances they keep on circulating and finally become trapped in the tissues of kidneys, lungs, skin, joints or blood vessels. The reaction of these complexes with complement results in inflammation and tissue damage.

(d) Immune deficiency diseases

Immune deficiency disorders occur due to the missing of one or more components of immune system, for example AIDS. **Causes** of immune deficiency diseases include:

1. Heredity.
2. Infection including viral infections such as influenza, infectious mono-nucleosis and measles.
3. Side effect of certain drugs used to treat patient of cancer or transplantation.
4. Blood transfusions, smoking, stress, surgery and malnutrition.
5. Antibodies not produced due to flaws in the B cell system
6. Lack of T cells due to missing or small and abnormal thymus.
7. Children born with poorly functioning immune systems.

HOSPITAL ACQUIRED INFECTIONS (NOSOCOMIAL INFECTIONS)

With the acceptance of the goal 'health for all' the role of hospitals in health care can be easily appreciated. On one hand hospitals are meant for treatment of diseases but on the other hand hospitals also represent an excellent place for transmission of infection. **Nosocomial** or hospital acquired (*nosocomium* = hospital) infection is an infection originating in a patient while in a hospital. It denotes a new disorder (unrelated to the patients primary condition) associated with being in a hospital. It includes infection acquired *in* the hospital but appearing *after* discharge and also such infections among the staff of the hospital. Examples include infection of surgical wounds, hepatitis B, urinary tract infections, and septicemia. One of the major problems of today in hospitals is the prevention of transmission of *Staphylococcus aureus* (the 'golden killer') in air, dust, and on fomites. Respiratory diseases like pneumonia, diphtheria, and scarlet fever are often transmitted by such means. Hospital infections may be due to ordinary risks or those peculiar to the environments of a hospital. Infections carried from one person to another are called **cross-infection**. Infections carried from one tissue to another in the same patient are called **auto-infections**. About 5–15% of hospital patients are affected by Nosocomial infections and about 90,000 people per year die of these infections.

(a) Factors involved in nosocomial infections

1. **Microorganisms in the hospital environment:** In spite of major efforts to control them, large numbers of pathogens live in hospitals. Common organisms include:

   (a) *Staphylococcus aureus*
   (b) *Escherichia coli*
   (c) *Pseudomonas aeruginosa.*

   Unfortunately, many of the strains of pathogens found in hospitals are resistant to antibiotics.

2. **Compromised host:** These are the patients weakened by other illnesses or conditions, including broken skin and a suppressed immune system. Invasive procedures such as anesthesia and surgery also increase the risk.

3. **Chain of transmission in the hospital:** a) direct contact transmission from hospital staff to patient, b) patient to patient, c) fomites, and d) ventilation system.

(b) Prevention of nosocomial infection

Hospitals are required to have an infection control committee, an infection control nurse, or an epidemiologist. Their job is to identify problem sources, check equipment for contamination, check sterilization procedures, etc.

Some means of controlling infection include:

1. Education of staff
2. Hand-washing and use of gloves
3. Aseptic techniques where appropriate
4. Careful handling of contaminated materials
5. Isolation, where appropriate.

Every year October 15th is practised worldwide as Global Hand Washing Day to create awareness about hand-washing as a measure to prevent infection.

Following **general measures** can be applied to **prevent Nosocomial infections**:

1. Patients of serious and easily transmissible diseases like tuberculosis, typhoid, and diphtheria should not be treated or nursed in open wards. They must be isolated.
2. Infants suffering from measles or whooping cough may be treated at home.
3. Isolation is also recommended for patients with *P. aeruginosa* or diarrhoeal infections or babies with *E. coli* infection and gastroenteritis.
4. Dressing of wounds should preferably be done in dressing room to minimize chances of cross-infection.
5. If new born babies need to be bathed, this should be done in stainless steel bowls, which can be easily cleaned and autoclaved (sterilized).
6. In general, isolation, hygiene and exclusion of carriers are most important preventive measures.

DISINFECTION

Our environment is full of microorganism (microbes). Some of these microbes are harmful, particularly those which cause infection. **Sterilization** is the process, which destroys and eliminates all microbes including spores. Disinfection is a less lethal process than sterilization. A **disinfectant** is a substance, which destroys infective microbes with the object of preventing transmission of disease. In the past disinfection was used only on in-animate (non-living) objects but it is now extended to include the skin and mucous membranes. An **antiseptic** is a substance that destroys or inhibits the growth of microbes. A disinfectant in low concentration can be used as antiseptic. Antiseptics are suitable for living tissues.

Disinfectants act by one or more of the following **mechanisms**:

1. Coagulation of bacteria cell protoplasm e.g. metallic salts and heat.
2. Oxidative burning of bacterial protoplasm e.g. $KMnO_4$.
3. Interference with metabolic processes of the microbes e.g. phenols.

A. Types of Disinfection

1. Concurrent disinfection

It refers to the application of disinfective measures as soon as possible after the discharge of infectious materials from the body of an infected person, or after the soiling of articles with such infectious discharges. Its aim is to prevent transmission of infection to doctors, nurses, medical attendant and neighbors, and disinfection of rooms. Throughout the course of an illness, materials like urine, faeces, vomit, contaminated linen, clothes, hands, dressing, apron, gloves etc are disinfected by concurrent disinfection. Thus further spread of infection is prevented.

2. Terminal disinfection

It is the disinfection of the infected material after removal of patient to hospital, after recovery or death. Rooms are disinfected by fumigation, floors and walls are sprayed with 2% formalin or 5% coal tar disinfectant or DDT, bedding and linen are disinfected by steam; and boots, leather goods etc are exposed to 3% formalin for 3 hours.

3. Prophylactic disinfection

It includes procedures like pasteurization of milk, chlorination of water, washing of hands and all aseptic techniques aiming at disrupting the pathway by which the microbes are transmitted.

B. Classification of Disinfectants

Different methods of disinfection are summarized in Fig. 9.5.

Natural agents

Direct and continuous exposure to ultraviolet (UV) rays of sunlight destroys

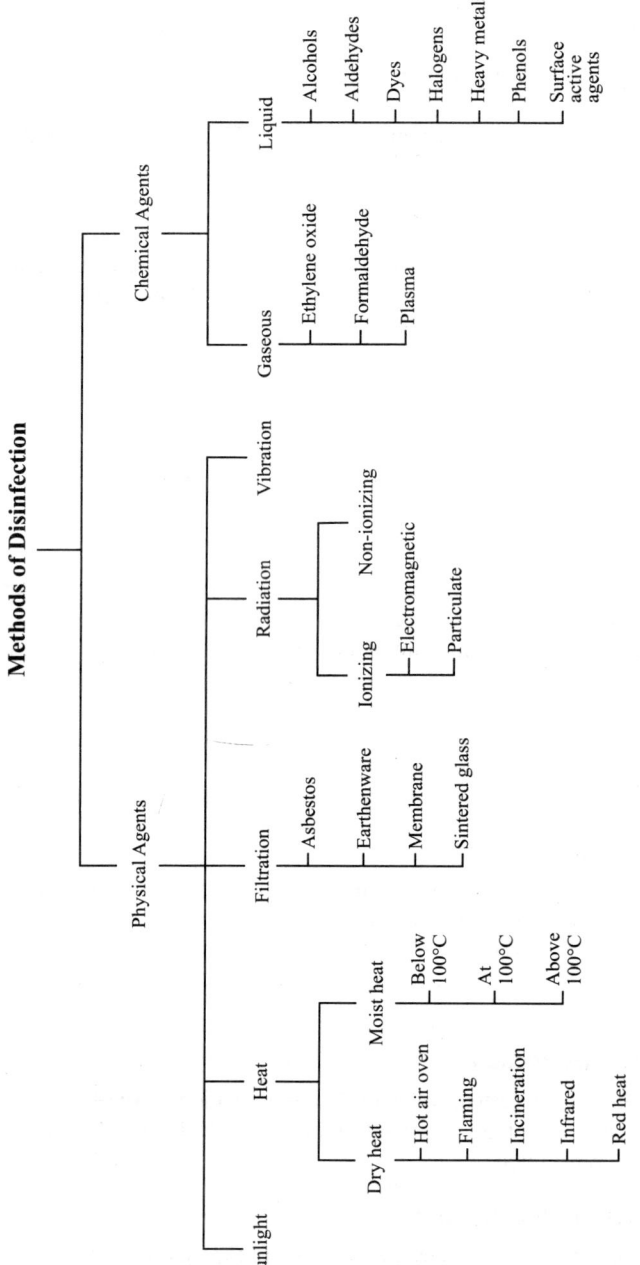

Fig. 9.5. Different methods of disinfection.

disease-producing organisms. Sunlight is not sporicidal, hence it does not sterilize.

Mechanism of action: The microbicidal activity of sunlight is mainly due to the presence of ultraviolet rays in it. It is responsible for spontaneous sterilization in natural conditions. In tropical countries, the sunlight is more effective in killing germs due to combination of ultraviolet rays and heat. Air causes drying or evaporation of moisture, which is lethal to most bacteria.

Articles disinfected: Linen, bedding and furniture may be disinfected by this method. By killing bacteria suspended in water, sunlight provides natural method of disinfection of water bodies such as tanks and lakes. Natural agents are not totally dependable for disinfection.

Physical agents

Burning or *incineration* is the most dependable method of disinfection of items of little value such as contaminated dressing, rags and towels. Faeces can also be disposed of by burning. Burning should be done in open air, preferably in an incinerator.

(a) Heat

Heat is considered to be most reliable method of disinfection of articles that can withstand heat. Those articles that cannot withstand high temperatures can still be operated at lower temperature by prolonging the duration of exposure.

Mechanism of action: Heat acts by oxidative effects as well as denaturation and coagulation of proteins.

(b) Dry heat

Mechanism of action: Dry heat acts by:
• Protein denaturation,
• Oxidative damage and toxic effects of elevated levels of electrolytes.

Red heat: Articles such as bacteriological loops, straight wires, tips of forceps, spatulas are treated by holding them in Bunsen flame till they become red hot. This is a simple method for effective sterilization of such articles, but is limited to those articles that can be heated to redness in flame.

Flaming: This is a method of passing the article over a Bunsen flame, but not heating it to redness. Articles such as scalpels, mouth of test tubes, flasks, glass slides and cover slips are passed through the flame a few times. Even though most vegetative cells are killed, there is no guarantee that spores too would die on such short exposure. This method too is limited to those articles that can be exposed to flame. Cracking of the glassware may occur.

Incineration: This is a method of destroying contaminated material by burning them in incinerator. Articles such as soiled dressings, animal carcasses, pathological material and bedding etc should be subjected to incineration. This technique results in the loss of the article, hence is suitable only for those articles that have to be disposed. Burning of polystyrene materials emits dense smoke, and hence they should not be incinerated.

Hot dry air (Hot air oven): It has no penetration power and hence does not kill spores. This method was introduced by Louis Pasteur. The method is useful for sterilization of articles like glassware, syringes, swabs, dressings, sharp instrument, oil etc. Sterilization is done at 16–180°C for 60 minutes in a hot air oven. The heat is transferred to the article by radiation, conduction and convection. The oven should be fitted with a thermostat control, temperature indicator, meshed shelves and must have adequate insulation. But many materials like plastic, rubber etc cannot withstand this temperature.

Infrared rays: Infrared rays bring about disinfection by generation of heat. Articles are placed in a moving conveyer belt and passed through a tunnel that is heated by infrared radiators to a temperature of 180°C. The articles are exposed to that temperature for a period of 7.5 minutes.

Articles disinfected: Metallic instruments (like forceps, scalpels and scissors), glassware (such as petri-dishes, pipettes, flasks, and all-glass syringes), swabs, oils, grease, petroleum jelly and some pharmaceutical products.

Advantages: It is an effective method of sterilization of heat stable articles. The articles remain dry after sterilization. This is the only method of sterilizing oils and powders.

Disadvantages:
1. Method is not suitable for materials, which cannot withstand high temperatures, for example plastics, rubber etc.
2. Since air is poor conductor of heat, hot air has poor penetration.
3. Cotton wool and paper may get slightly charred.
4. Glasses may become smoky.
5. Takes longer time compared to autoclave.

(c) Moist heat

Boiling is an effective method of disinfection. Boiling for 1 to 15 minutes kills most of the bacteria but spores cannot be killed by boiling for 3 minutes. The method can be used for disinfection of small instrument, knives, gloves etc. Boiling for about 3 minutes is sufficient for disinfecting the linen, utensils and bedpans. Moist heat is superior to dry heat in action. Temperature required to kill microbe by dry heat is more than the moist heat.

Mechanism of action: Moist heat acts by coagulation and denaturation of proteins.

At temperature below 100°C (Pasteurization): This process was originally employed by Louis Pasteur. Currently this procedure is employed in food and dairy industry. There are two methods of pasteurization, the *holder method* (heating at 63°C for 3 minutes) and *flash method* (heating at 72°C for 15 seconds) followed by quick cooling to 13°C. Other pasteurization methods include Ultra-High Temperature (UHT), 140°C for 15 seconds and 149°C for

0.5 second. This method is suitable to destroy most milk-borne pathogens like Salmonella, Mycobacteria, Streptococci, Staphylococci and Brucella, however Coxiella may survive pasteurization. Efficacy is tested by phosphatase test and methylene blue test.

At temperature above 100°C (Autoclaving): Autoclaving is a method of sterilization using saturated steam and is one of the most efficient methods. It works on the principle of household pressure cooker. Water boils at 100°C at atmospheric pressure, but if pressure is raised, the temperature at which the water boils also increases. In an autoclave the water is boiled in a closed chamber. As the pressure rises, the boiling point of water also raises. A temperature of 121°C at 15 lb pressure for 15 minutes kills all the micro-organisms because of the greater penetration power of the saturated steam. It is most effective method for sterilization of linen, dressing, gloves, syringe, certain instrument and culture media.

Chemical agents

Chemical disinfectants are those chemicals, which can destroy pathogenic bacteria from inanimate surfaces. Some chemicals have very narrow spectrum of activity and some have very wide. Those chemicals that can be safely applied over skin and mucus membranes are called *antiseptics*. Chemical disinfectants have wider range of application than physical agents. Articles which cannot be easily disinfected by physical agents can be disinfected by chemical agents.

Mechanism of action: They act by oxidizing and coagulating the protoplasm of bacteria.

Ideal disinfectant

Requirements of an ideal disinfectant are as follows:

1. It should have a great penetration power.
2. It should have a powerful and rapid germicidal action.
3. It should have definite efficiency for a particular type of organisms.
4. It should be stable in presence of organic matter and must retain activity in the presence of stool and urine.
5. It should not be injurious to human tissue or the material to be disinfected.
6. It should mix in water in all proportions and form a uniform emulsion.
7. It should be cheap and easily available.
8. It should be neither toxic nor caustic in action and devoid of unpleasant odor.
9. It should have wide spectrum of activity.
10. It should be able to destroy microbes within practical period of time.
11. It should make effective contact and be wettable.
12. It should be active in any pH, stable and have long shelf-life.
13. It should be non-toxic, non-allergenic, non-irritative or non-corrosive.
14. It should not leave non-volatile residue or stain.
15. Its efficacy should not be lost on reasonable dilution.
16. It should not be expensive and must be available easily.

Such an ideal disinfectant is not yet available. The level of disinfection achieved depends on contact time, temperature, type and concentration of the active ingredient, the presence of organic matter, the type and quantum of microbial load.

Classification of chemical disinfectants

1. **Based on consistency:**
   (a) Liquid (examples – alcohols, aldehydes, phenols, halogens, heavy metals, surface active agents, dyes, hydrogen peroxide, β-propiolactone).
   (b) Gaseous (examples – formaldehyde vapor, ethylene oxide).
2. **Based on spectrum of activity:**
   (a) High level: Active against vegetative cells, mycobacteria, spores, fungi, viruses, etc (examples – ethylene oxide, gluteraldehyde, formaldehyde).
   (b) Intermediate level: This includes phenolics and halogens, which are active against vegetative cells, mycobacteria, fungi and viruses but inactive against spores.
   (c) Low level: Alcohols, quaternary ammonium compounds, which are active against vegetative cells and fungi but inactive against spores and mycobacteria.
3. **Based on mechanism of action:**
   (a) Action on membrane (examples – alcohol, detergent).
   (b) Denaturation of cellular proteins (examples – alcohol, phenol).
   (c) Oxidation of essential sulphydryl groups of enzymes (examples – H_2O_2, halogens).
   (d) Alkylation of amino-, carboxyl- and hydroxyl-group (examples – ethylene oxide, formaldehyde)
   (e) Damage to nucleic acids (examples – ethylene oxide, formaldehyde)

Some important chemical disinfectants are discussed below.

(i) Alcohols

Mode of action: Alcohols dehydrate cells, disrupt membranes and cause coagulation of protein, for example ethyl alcohol, isopropyl alcohol and methyl alcohol.

Applications:
1. A 70% aqueous solution is more effective at killing microbes than absolute alcohols.
2. 70% ethyl alcohol (spirit) is used as antiseptic on skin.
3. Isopropyl alcohol is used to disinfect clinical thermometers.
4. Methyl alcohol kills fungal spores, hence is useful in disinfecting inoculation hoods.

Disadvantages: Skin irritant, volatile (evaporates rapidly), inflammable.

(ii) Aldehydes

Mode of action: Act through alkylation of amino-, carboxyl- or hydroxyl-group, and probably damage nucleic acids. Aldehydes kill all microorganisms, including spores, for example formaldehyde and gluteraldehyde.

Applications:
1. 40% formaldehyde (formalin) is used for surface disinfection and fumigation of rooms, chambers, operation theatres, biological safety cabinets, wards, sick rooms etc. Fumigation is achieved by boiling formalin, heating paraformaldehyde or treating formalin with potassium permanganate. It also sterilizes bedding, furniture and books. 10% formalin with 0.5% tetraborate sterilizes clean metal instruments.
2. Gluteraldehyde (2%) is used to sterilize thermometers, cystoscopes, bronchoscopes, centrifuges, anasethetic equipments etc. An exposure of at least 3 hours at alkaline pH is required for action by gluteraldehyde.
3. 2% formaldehyde at 40°C for 2 minutes is used to disinfect wool and 0.25% at 60°C for six hours to disinfect animal hair and bristles.

Disadvantages:
1. Vapours are irritating (must be neutralized by ammonia).
2. Has poor penetration.
3. Leaves non-volatile residue.
4. Activity is reduced in the presence of protein.
5. Gluteraldehyde requires alkaline pH and only those articles that are wettable can be sterilized.

(iii) Phenols

Mode of action: Phenols act by disruption of membranes, precipitation of proteins and inactivation of enzymes, for example 5% phenol, 1–5% Cresol, 5% Lysol (a saponified cresol), hexachlorophene, chlorhexidine, chloroxylenol (Dettol).

Applications:
1. Phenols are coal-tar derivatives. They act as disinfectants at high concentration and as antiseptics at low concentrations.
2. They are bactericidal, fungicidal and mycobactericidal but are inactive against spores and most viruses.
3. They are not readily inactivated by organic matter.
4. The corrosive phenolics are used for disinfection of ward floors, in discarding jars in laboratories and disinfection of bedpans.
5. Chlorhexidine can be used in an isopropanol solution for skin disinfection, or as an aqueous solution for wound irrigation. It is often used as an antiseptic hand wash.
6. 20% Chlorhexidine gluconate solution is used for preoperative hand and skin preparation and for general skin disinfection. Chlorhexidine gluconate is also mixed with quaternary ammonium compounds such as cetrimide to get stronger and broader antimicrobial effects (example, Savlon).

7. Chloroxylenols cause less irritation, hence can be used for topical purposes and are more effective against Gram positive bacteria than Gram negative bacteria.
8. Hexachlorophene is chlorinated diphenyl, which causes much less irritation. It has marked effect over Gram positive bacteria but poor effect over Gram negative bacteria, mycobacteria, fungi and viruses.
9. Triclosan is organic phenyl ether with good activity against Gram positive bacteria and effective to some extent against many Gram negative bacteria including Pseudomonas. It also has fair activity on fungi and viruses.

Limitations:
1. Toxic
2. Corrosive
3. Skin irritant
4. Chlorhexidine is inactivated by anionic soaps.
5. Chloroxylenol is inactivated by hard water.

(iv) Halogens

Mode of action: They are oxidizing agents and cause damage by oxidation of essential sulphydryl groups of enzymes. Chlorine reacts with water to form hypochlorous acid, which is microbicidal, for example chlorine compounds (chlorine, bleach, hypo chlorite) and iodine compounds (tincture iodine, iodophores).

Applications:
1. Tincture of iodine (2% iodine in 70% alcohol) is an antiseptic.
2. Iodine can be combined with neutral carrier polymers such as polyvinylpyrrolidone to prepare iodophores such as Povidone-Iodine.
3. Iodophores permit slow release and reduce the irritation of the antiseptic. For hand washing iodophores are diluted in 50% alcohol.
4. 10% Povidone Iodine is used undiluted in pre- and post-operative skin disinfection.
5. Chlorine gas is used to bleach water. Household bleach can be used to disinfect floors. Household bleach is used in a stock dilution of 1 : 10. In higher concentrations chlorine is used to disinfect swimming pools.
6. 0.5% sodium hypochlorite is used in serology and virology. It is also used at a dilution of 1 : 1 in decontamination of infectious material.
7. Mercuric chloride is used as a disinfectant.

Disadvantages:
1. They are rapidly inactivated in the presence of organic matter.
2. Iodine is corrosive and staining.
3. Bleach solution is corrosive and will corrode stainless steel surfaces.

(v) Heavy metals

Mode of action: Heavy metals act by precipitation of proteins and oxidation of sulphydryl groups. They are bacteriostatic, for example mercuric chloride, silver nitrate, copper sulfate, organic mercury salts such as mercurochrome, merthiolate.

Applications:
1. Silver sulphadiazine is used topically to prevent colonization and infection of burn tissues.
2. Mercurials are active against viruses at dilution of 1 : 50 to 1 : 1,000.
3. Merthiolate at a concentration of 1 : 10,00 is used in preservation of serum.
4. Copper salts are used as fungicide.

Limitations:
1. Readily inactivated by organic matter.
2. Mercuric chloride is highly toxic.

(vi) Surface active agents

These are soaps or detergents, which could be anionic or cationic.

Detergents containing negatively charged long chain hydrocarbon are called *anionic detergents* such as soaps and bile salts.

If the fat-soluble part is made to have a positive charge by combining with a quaternary nitrogen atom, it is called *cationic detergents* which are known as quaternary ammonium compounds; examples include cetrimide and benzalkonium chloride.

Mechanism of action: Surface active agents have long chain hydrocarbons that are fat soluble and charged ions that are water-soluble. Hence, they concentrate at interfaces between lipid containing membrane of bacterial cell and surrounding aqueous medium. They disrupt membrane resulting in leakage of cell constituents.

Applications:
1. They are active against vegetative cells, mycobacteria and enveloped viruses.
2. They are widely used as disinfectants at dilution of 1–2% for domestic use and in hospitals.

Limitations:
1. Their activity is reduced by hard water, anionic detergents and organic matter.
2. Pseudomonas can metabolize cetrimide, using them as a carbon, nitrogen and energy source.

(vii) Dyes

Action against microbes: They are more effective against Gram positive bacteria than Gram negative bacteria and are more bacteriostatic in action. Acridine dyes are bactericidal because of their interaction with bacterial nucleic acids. Ethidium bromide intercalates between base pairs in DNA; for example aniline dyes, crystal violet, malachite green and brilliant green; acridine dyes such as acriflavin and aminacrine; and ethidium bromide.

Applications:
1. They may be used topically as antiseptics to treat mild burns.
2. They are used as paint on the skin to treat bacterial skin infections.
3. The dyes are used as selective agents in certain selective media.

(viii) Hydrogen peroxide

Mode of action: It acts on the microorganisms through its release of nascent oxygen. Hydrogen peroxide produces hydroxyl-free radical that damages proteins and DNA.

Applications:
1. It is used at 6% concentration to decontaminate the instruments, and equipments such as ventilators.
2. 3% Hydrogen Peroxide Solution is used for skin disinfection and deodorising wounds and ulcers. Strong solutions are sporicidal.

(ix) Ethylene oxide (EO)

It is a cyclic molecule, which is a colorless liquid at room temperature. It has a sweet ethereal odor, readily polymerizes and is flammable. Efficiency testing is done using *Bacillus subtilis* var niger.

Mode of action: It is an alkylating agent. It acts by alkylating sulphydryl-, amino-, carboxyl- and hydroxyl-groups.

Applications:
1. It is a highly effective chemi-sterilant, capable of killing spores rapidly.
2. It has good penetration and is well absorbed by porous material. Since it is highly flammable, it is usually combined with CO_2 (10% CO_2 + 90% EO) or dichlorodifluoromethane. It requires presence of humidity.
3. It is used to sterilize heat-labile articles such as bedding, textiles, rubber, plastics, syringes, disposable petri dishes, and complex apparatus like heart-lung machine, respiratory and dental equipments.

Disadvantages:
1. It is highly toxic.
2. Irritating to eyes and skin.
3. Highly flammable.
4. Mutagenic and carcinogenic.

(x) β-Propiolactone (BPL)

It is a colorless liquid with pungent to slightly sweetish smell. It is a condensation product of ketane with formaldehyde.

Mode of action: It is an alkylating agent and acts through alkylation of carboxyl- and hydroxyl-groups.

Applications:
1. It is an effective sporicidal agent, and has broad-spectrum activity.
2. 0.2% is used to sterilize biological products.

3. It is more efficient in fumigation than formaldehyde.
4. It is used to sterilize vaccines, tissue grafts, surgical instruments and enzymes.

Disadvantages: It has poor penetrating power and is a carcinogen.

PHYSICOCHEMICAL METHODS

Mode of action: A physicochemical method cpmbines both physical and chemical method. Use of steam-formaldehyde is a physiochemical method of sterilization, which takes into account action of steam as well as that of formaldehyde. Saturated steam at a pressure of 263 mm Hg has a temperature of 70°C. The air is removed from the autoclave chamber and saturated steam at sub-atmospheric pressure is flushed in. Formaldehyde is then injected with steam in a series of pulses, each of 5-1 minutes. The articles are held at this holding temperature for one hour. Formaldehyde is then flushed by inflow of steam.

Disadvantages: Condensation of formaldehyde occurs and induction of large volume of formaldehyde wets the steam resulting in loss of latent heat.

Commonly Used Disinfectants

Coaltar derivatives: Phenol (carbolic acid) was the first antiseptic used by Joseph Lister in 1865. It is used as a standard to compare the activity of other disinfectant. Pure phenol is not an effective disinfectant. Crude phenol is a mixture of phenol and cresol that is commonly used for disinfection. It acts against Gram postive and Gram negative bacteria and certain viruses. A 5% solution is bactericidal and kills all vegetative bacteria and some spores. A dilute solution (1 : 1000) is bacteriostatic. Most important use of phenol is in disinfecting faeces and sputum or any other organic matter. It is not harmful to metal or cloth. It can cause severe burns to the skin and can also cause toxic reactions.

Cresol is thrice as powerful as phenol. It is used as 5 to 10% solution for disinfection of rooms, latrines, excreta, sputum, drains etc. *Saponified Cresol* is the cresol emulsified with soap; two examples are Lysol and Cylin. They are powerful disinfectants.

Lysol contains 5 to 60% cresol. It has greater antiseptic action but less poisonous than phenol or cresol. It is used as 1% solution for hands, 2% solution for cloths, floors and 5% solution for excreta, sputum etc. It is especially useful for disinfection of table tops, floors, walls, rectal thermometer and articles contaminated with tubercle bacilli.

Cyllin is cheaper and powerful disinfectant for privies and drains. A 1 : 16 solution destroys streptococci in a few hours. For general purpose it is used as a 1 : 5 dilution. The drawbacks of this disinfectant are that it stains linen and is caustic to the skin.

Phenyl is a crude mixture of phenol and cresol. It is cheap and useful as 5 to 10% solution.

Chlorohexidine (Hibitane) is a popular antiseptic, highly active against vegetative Gram positive organism. 0.5% solution can be used as effective hand lotion. Creams and lotions containing 1% chlorohexidine are recommended for burns and hand disinfection. It is expensive but has found wide use as it can be mixed with other disinfectant such as Salvon.

Hexachlorophene is highly active against Gram positive organisms. It is used in 1 to 3% concentration for the pre-operative scrubbing of surgeons and pre- and post-operative skin preparation of the patients. It is slow in action.

Detergent: All detergents are not disinfectants but several compounds combine the properties of detergent, surface tension reducers and disinfectants. They are non-poisonous and non-irritating to the skin and mucous membranes but are expensive and not effective against spores.

Cetrimide is a quaternary ammonium compound used as a 1% solution for antiseptic action. It actively kills vegetative Gram positive bacteria. It is manufactured under the trade name 'Cetavlon'.

Savlon is a combination of Cetavlon and Hibitane. A 1 : 3 dilution in alcohol destroys vegetative bacteria in 1 to 2 minutes; a 1 : 6 dilution in alcohol disinfects clinical thermometers within 3 minutes.

Dettol (Chloroxylenol) is quite popular as a skin/wound disinfectant in many household. It is relatively non-toxic and can be safely used in high concentration. It is easily inactivated by organic matter. It is active against streptococci but some Gram positive bacteria like *P. aureus* can actually grow in a Dettol solution. Instrument and plastic equipment can be disinfected in 5% Dettol solution in about 2 minutes. It is inactivated by hard water and organic matter.

DISINFECTION PROCEDURES

(a) Faeces and Urine

Faeces and urine can be disinfected in many ways. These should be collected in impervious vessels, mixed with one of the following disinfectant and allowed to remain in contact for the prescribed number of hours.

Disinfectant	Concentration	Contact period
Cresol	3–10% solution	1–2 hours
Lysol	5% solution	1–2 hours
Phenol	10% solution	1–2 hours
Bleaching powder	8%	1–2 hours
Milk of Lime	Mix 2 volumes of disinfectant with 1 volume of faeces/urine	4 hours

If no disinfectant is available then a bucket of boiling water can be added to faeces, covered and allowed to stand until cool. The disinfected material must be emptied into water closet or buried in ground.

(b) Sputum

Sputum should be collected on paper handkerchiefs or gauze, which is destroyed by burning or by autoclaving at 2 lb pressure for 2 minutes or by boiling. Phenol (10%) is especially useful to disinfect sputum. A 3 to 10% solution of Cresol or 5% solution of Lysol or bleaching powder are also useful.

(c) Room

Gaseous disinfection (fumigation) is the easiest and the best method. Formaldehyde vapor is the most suitable disinfectant for rooms. Formaldehyde does not affect metal or colored materials and is an irritant. Form-o-chloral is obtained by heating formalin under pressure with a little calcium carbonate solution. 0.5 litre of Form-o-chloral is sufficient for 100 cu ft. space. Alternatively 14 g of $KMnO_4$ crystals are taken and 0.5 litre of formalin plus equal volume of water are poured over it. This is kept in room for 6 hours for effective disinfection of 100 cu ft. area. The formaldehyde gas is most effective at a high temperature and a relative humidity of 8 to 90%. A 100cu ft. space can also be disinfected by heating 25 tablets of Paraform in Alphorment lamp. 0.9 kg bleaching powder + 1 liter of formalin can disinfect 100 cu ft. space. Chlorine is also a good disinfectant and deodorant but it is irritating. It is used as 1 g bleaching powder + 0.5 kg H_2SO_4 or HCl for 100 cu ft. area. A hot mixture (8 parts of NaCl + 2 parts of MnO_2 + 2 parts of H_2SO_4 + 2 parts of water) is also suitable for 100 cu ft. space. Chloropicrine 2ml liquid per cu ft. space also acts as a disinfectant.

Besides these disinfection procedures, it is recommended that the rooms should be regularly cleaned, properly ventilated for airing and exposed to sunlight. Phenol can be used for mopping floors, walls etc. A 2% solution of Lysol can be used for disinfection of floors; white-washing of walls and roofs with lime is also useful. Floors and walls can also be sprayed with 2% formaldehyde or 5% coaltar or DDT.

(d) Linen

Linen is best disinfected by UV rays of the sun, which kill bacteria. Blankets, pillows and mattresses can be disinfected by this method. Formaldehyde gas can also be used for disinfection of blankets and beddings, which cannot be boiled. Ionizing radiations (gamma radiation) are particularly suitable for disinfection of linen but it is an expensive method. Other types of linen can be disinfected by boiling in disinfectant solution.

(e) Instruments

3 to 10% solution of Cresol can disinfect knives. Clinical thermometers can be disinfected by 1 : 6 parts of Savlon in spirit for 3 minutes. Rectal thermometers contaminated with tubercle bacilli can be disinfected with Lysol. A 0.25–3% solution of Amphyl (a phenolic compound) is suitable for surgical instruments. A freshly prepared solution of sodium hypochlorite containing 10 to 20 ppm

of available chlorine has been recommended for sterilization of infants feeding bottles.

(f) Dead bodies

Dead bodies of the persons who suffered from infectious diseases can be a source of infection and hence their handling requires special precautions. They should be wrapped and treated with powerful disinfectants. Cremation or burial should be done without delay.

Pharmacists should be thoroughly familiar with the methods of disinfection and evaluation of disinfectants.

Glossary

Agent Anything that can cause a disease is known as agent. It is a factor, such as a microorganism, chemical substance, or form of radiation, whose presence, excessive presence, or relative absence is essential for the occurrence of a disease.

Airborne disease The transmission of disease causing microorganisms through the air to the human respiratory tract (e.g. nose, mouth, throat, and lungs).

Allergen Any substance that causes an allergy.

Antibiotics Substances produced by one microbe that inhibits or kills another microbe. Often the term is used more generally to include synthetic and semisynthetic antimicrobial agents.

Antibody A molecule (also known an immunoglobulin) produced by a mature B cell (plasma cell) in response to an antigen. When an antibody attaches to an antigen, it helps the body destroy or inactivate the antigen.

Antigen A substance or molecule that is recognized by the immune system. The antigen can be from foreign origin such as bacteria or viruses.

Antimicrobial drugs Substances that kill or prevent the spreading of infectious agents or organisms in order to prevent the spread of infection.

Antisepsis The use of chemicals (antiseptics) to make skin or mucus membranes devoid of pathogenic microorganisms.

Antiserum A serum rich in antibodies against a particular microbe.

Appendix Lymphoid organ in the intestine.

Asepsis The employment of techniques (such as usage of gloves, air filters, UV rays etc) to achieve microbe-free environment.

Asymptomatic carriers A person or animal not currently showing the symptoms of a communicable disease but that can serve as a potential source of infection.

Asymptomatic A term used to describe an individual who does not currently show symptoms of the disease but who, in fact, may be infected. Asymptomatic individuals may develop symptoms of the disease at a later point in time if and when the disease onsets.

Autoantibody An antibody that reacts against a person's own tissue.

Autoimmune disease Disease that results when the immune system mistakenly attacks the body's own tissues. Examples include multiple sclerosis, type 1 diabetes, rheumatoid arthritis, and systemic lupus erythematosus.

B cell (B lymphocyte) A small white blood cell crucial to the immune defences. B cells come from bone marrow and develop into blood cells called plasma cells, which are the source of antibodies.

Bacteria Microscopic organisms composed of a single cell. Some cause disease.

Bacterial disease Infections and associated diseases caused by bacteria, general or unspecified.

Bactericidal Chemical that can kill or inactivate bacteria. Depending on the spectrum of activity such chemicals may be called as bactericidal, virucidal, fungicidal, microbicidal, sporicidal, tuberculocidal or germicidal.

Bacteriostasis A condition where the multiplication of the bacteria is inhibited without killing them.

Basophil A white blood cell that contributes to inflammatory reactions. Along with mast cells, basophils are responsible for the symptoms of allergy.

Blood vessel An artery, vein, or capillary that carries blood to and from the heart and body tissues.

Carrier host A person or animal without apparent disease that harbours a specific infectious agent and is capable of transmitting the agent to others. The carrier state may be of short or long duration (transient carrier or chronic carrier).

Carrier A person or animal that harbours a specific infectious agent without discernible clinical disease and serves as a potential source of infection.

Cell The smallest unit of life; the basic living unit that makes up tissues.

Chronic disease Any illness is called "chronic" if it is long-lasting or even lifelong. The opposite of chronic is "acute", referring to diseases that come on quickly and often do not last long (if they last, they are said to become "chronic").

Clone A group of genetically identical cells or organisms descended from a single common ancestor; or, to reproduce identical copies.

Communicable disease (*syn.* Infectious disease) An illness due to a specific infectious agent or its toxic products that is transmitted from an infected person, animal, or inanimate reservoir to a susceptible host.

Complement A complex series of blood proteins whose action "complements" the work of antibodies. Complement destroys bacteria, produces inflammation, and regulates immune reactions.

Contact A person or animal that has had an opportunity to acquire an infection by being within the environment of an infected individual.

Contagious Capable of transmitting disease.

Contaminated Impure or unclean because of contact with a communicable disease agent.

Contraceptive A device, drug, or chemical agent that prevents conception and, in some instances, may help prevent the spread of a sexually transmitted disease.

Cytokines Powerful chemical substances secreted by cells that enable the body's cells to communicate with one another. Cytokines include lymphokines produced by lymphocytes and monokines produced by monocytes and macrophages.

Decontamination The process of removal of contaminating pathogenic microorganisms from the articles by a process of sterilization or disinfection. It is the use of physical or chemical means to remove, inactivate, or destroy living organisms on a surface so that the organisms are no longer infectious.

Diagnosis The act or process of identifying or determining the nature and cause of a disease or injury through evaluation of patient history, examination, and review of laboratory data. Also, the opinion derived from such an evaluation.

Disinfection The process of elimination of most pathogenic microorganisms (excluding bacterial spores) on inanimate objects. Disinfection can be achieved by physical or chemical methods. Chemicals used in disinfection are called disinfectants. Different disinfectants have different target ranges, not all disinfectants can kill all microorganisms. Some methods of disinfection such as filtration do not kill bacteria, they separate them out. Sterilization is an absolute condition while disinfection is not. The two are not synonymous.

DNA (deoxyribonucleic acid) A long molecule found in the cell nucleus. Molecules of DNA carry the cell's genetic information.

Dormant A virus that is inactive in an infected individual or animal but may reactivate given the right circumstances.

Droplet nuclei The residue of dried droplets that may remain suspended in the air for long periods, may be blown over great distances, and are easily inhaled into the lungs and exhaled.

Enteric diseases Diseases of or relating to the intestines; "intestinal disease".

Environmental factors An extrinsic factor (insects, geology, climate, sanitation, health services, etc.) which affects the agent and the opportunity for exposure. Anything not agent but outside factors influencing exposure of infection is considered as environmental factors.

Enzyme A protein produced by living cells that promotes the chemical processes of life without itself being altered.

Eosinophil A white blood cell containing granules filled with chemicals damaging to parasites and enzymes that affect inflammatory reactions.

Epithelial cells Cells that make up the epithelium, the covering for internal and external body surfaces.

Exposure To have contact with an infectious disease agent or its toxic products.

Faeces (syn. Stool) The medical and scientific term for the 'excrement discharged from the intestines.'

Foodborne illness (*syn.* Food poisoning) Any illness resulting from the consumption of food contaminated with pathogenic bacteria, toxins, viruses, prions, or parasites.

Fungus A member of a class of relatively primitive vegetable organisms. Fungi include mushrooms, yeasts, rusts, molds, and smuts.

Gene A unit of genetic material (DNA) inherited from a parent that controls specific characteristics. Genes carry coded directions a cell uses to make specific proteins that perform specific functions.

Genome A full set of genes in a person or any other living thing.

Genotype The genetic makeup encoded in DNA.

Graft rejection An immune response against transplanted tissue.

Granulocyte A phagocytic white blood cell filled with granules, for example neutrophils, eosinophils, basophils, and mast cells.

Growth factors Chemicals secreted by cells that stimulate proliferation of/or changes in the physical properties of other cells.

Helper T cells (Th cells) A subset of T cells that carry the CD4 surface marker and are essential for turning on antibody production, activating cytotoxic T cells, and initiating many other immune functions.

Hepatitis The name of several viruses that cause liver diseases including hepatitis A, hepatitis B, and hepatitis C.

Histocompatibility testing A test conducted before transplant operations to find a donor whose MHC molecules are similar to the recipient's; helps reduce the strength of transplant rejection.

HIV (Human immunodeficiency virus) The virus that causes AIDS.

Host A person or other living organism that can be infected by an infectious agent under natural conditions and sometimes experimental conditions.

Iatrogenic Refers to adverse effects or complications caused by or resulting from medical treatment or advice. In addition to harmful consequences of actions by physicians, iatrogenesis can also refer to actions by other healthcare professionals, such as psychologist, therapist, pharmacists, nurses, dentist etc.

Immune response Reaction of the immune system to foreign substances. Although normal immune responses are designed to protect the body from pathogens, immune dys-regulation can damage normal cells and tissues, as in the case of autoimmune diseases.

Immune system The system (including the thymus and bone marrow and lymphoid tissues) that protects the body from foreign substances and pathogenic organisms by producing the immune response.

Immunizations (*syn.* Vaccination, Shot) The administration of a weakened or killed form of a disease-causing agent to induce the body's immune system to produce antibodies against the disease, in the event of a future exposure to the specific disease-causing agent.

Immunoglobulin One of a family of large protein molecules, also known as antibodies, produced by mature B cells (plasma cells).

Immunosuppressive Capable of reducing immune responses.

Incidence rate The number of new cases of a specified disease during a defined period of time, divided by the number of persons in a stated population in which the cases occurred. This is usually expressed as cases per 1,000 or 100,000 per year. This rate may be expressed as age- or gender-specific or as specific for any other population characteristic or subdivision.

Incubation period The time interval between contact with an infectious agent and onset of symptoms of disease.

Infectious disease A clinically manifested illness of humans or animals resulting from an infection.

Infectious period The length of time that a person or animal harbouring a communicable disease is able to transmit that disease to another person or animal.

Infectivity The proportion of persons exposed to a causative agent who become infected by an infectious disease.

Inflammation An immune system reaction to 'foreign' invaders such as microbes or allergens. Symptoms include redness, swelling, pain, or heat.

Inflammatory response Redness, warmth, and swelling produced in response to infection; the result of increased blood flow and an influx of immune cells and their secretions.

Innate An immune system function that is inborn and provides an all-purpose defence against invasion by microbes.

Interferon A protein produced by cells that stimulates antivirus immune responses or alters the physical properties of immune cells.

Interleukins A major group of lymphokines and monokines.

Lymph node A small bean-shaped organ of the immune system, distributed widely throughout the body and linked by lymphatic vessels. Lymph nodes are garrisons of B and T cells, dendritic cells, macrophages, and other kinds of immune cells.

Lymph A transparent, slightly yellow fluid that carries lymphocytes, bathes the body tissues, and drains into the lymphatic vessels.

Lymphatic vessels Network of channels throughout body, similar to the blood vessels, which transport lymph to the immune organs and into the bloodstream.

Lymphocyte A small white blood cell produced in the lymphoid organs and essential to immune defences. B cells, T cells, and NK T cells are lymphocytes.

Lymphoid organ An organ of the immune system where lymphocytes develop and congregate. These organs include the bone marrow, thymus, lymph nodes, spleen, and various other clusters of lymphoid tissue. Blood vessels and lymphatic vessels are also lymphoid organs.

Macrophage A large and versatile immune cell that devours invading pathogens and other intruders. Macrophages stimulate other immune cells by presenting them with small pieces of the invaders.

Major histocompatibility complex (MHC) A group of genes that controls several aspects of the immune response. MHC genes code for "self" markers on all body cells.

Malaise A vague feeling of bodily discomfort, as at the beginning of an illness.

Memory cells A subset of T cells and B cells that have been exposed to antigens and can then respond more readily when the immune system encounters those same antigens again.

Microbe or microorganism A microscopic living organism; examples include bacteria, protozoa, and some fungi and parasites. Viruses are also called microbes.

Molecule The smallest amount of a specific chemical substance. Large molecules such as proteins, fats, carbohydrates, and nucleic acids are the building blocks of a cell, and a gene determines how each molecule is produced.

Monoclonal antibody An antibody produced by a single B cell or its identical progeny that is specific for a given antigen. Monoclonal antibodies are used as research tools for binding to specific protein molecules, and are invaluable in research, medicine, and industry.

Monocyte A large phagocytic white blood cell which, upon entering tissue, develops into a macrophage.

Morbidity The number person affected by a disease.

Mortality The death rate caused by a disease.

Natural killer (NK) cell A large granule-containing lymphocyte that recognizes and kills cells lacking self antigens. These cells' target recognition molecules are different from T cells.

Neutrophil A white blood cell that is an abundant and important phagocyte.

NK T cell A T cell that has some characteristics of NK cells. It produces large amounts of cytokines when stimulated, and is activated by fatty substances (lipids) bound to non-MHC molecules called CD1d.

Organ A part of the body that has a specific function, such as the lungs.

Organism An individual living being composed of one or more cells.

Outbreak The occurrence of cases of a disease or condition in any area over a given period of time in excess of the expected number of cases.

Parasite A plant or animal that lives, grows, and feeds on or within another living organism.

Passive immunity Immunity resulting from the transfer of antibodies or antiserum produced by another person.

Pathogen A disease-causing organism or virus.

Phagocyte A large white blood cell that contributes to immune defences by ingesting microbes or other cells and foreign particles.

Phagocytosis Process by which one cell engulfs another cell or large particle.

Plasma cell A large antibody-producing cell that develops from B cells.

Platelet A cellular fragment critical for blood clotting and sealing off wounds.

Portal of entry To gain entry to the body, pathogens must either (1) infect cells in one of the body surfaces (skin, respiratory mucosa, alimentary tract), (2) otherwise breach the surface (by trauma, bite, or injection), or (3) be transmitted congenitally.

Prevalence rate The total number of persons sick or portraying a certain condition in a stated population at a particular time (point prevalence), or during a stated period of time (period prevalence), regardless of when that illness or condition began, divided by the population at risk of having the disease or condition at the point in time or midway through the period in which they occurred.

Recurrence The concept that an illness may come back again.

Reservoir of disease A reservoir of disease is any person, animal, or thing (fomite) which can contain the cause of a disease without suffering from it.
   Reservoir means any person, animal, arthropod, plant, soil or substance (or combination of these) in which an infectious agent normally lives and multiplies, on which it depends primarily for survival, and where it reproduces itself in such manner that it can be transmitted to a susceptible host.

Sanitization The process of chemical or mechanical cleansing, applicable in public health systems. Usually used by the food industry. It reduces microbes on eating utensils to safe, acceptable levels for public health.

Serum The clear liquid that separates from the blood when it is allowed to clot. Serum contains the antibodies that were present in the whole blood.

Sexually-transmitted disease (STD) (*syn*. **Venereal disease**) A group of various diseases that are spread by sexual contact.

Sterilization The process where all the living microorganisms, including bacterial spores are killed. Sterilization can be achieved by physical, chemical and physiochemical means.

Strain The type or subtype of a bacteria or virus.

Surveillance Surveillance of disease is the continuing scrutiny of all aspects of occurrence and spread of a disease that are pertinent to effective control.

Symptomatic A term used to describe an individual who shows symptoms of a disease.

T cell (T lymphocyte) A small white blood cell that recognizes antigen fragments bound to cell surfaces by specialized antibody-like receptors. 'T' stands for the thymus gland, where T cells develop and acquire their receptors.

T cell receptor Complex protein molecule on the surfaces of T cells that recognizes bits of foreign antigen bound to self-MHC molecules.

Tissue A group of similar cells joined to perform the same function.

Tolerance A state of immune non-responsiveness to a particular antigen or group of antigens.

Toxin An agent produced in plants and bacteria, normally very damaging to cells.

Transmission of infection Any mode or mechanism by which an infectious agent is spread through the environment or to another person.

Transmission Any mechanism by which an infectious agent is spread from a source or reservoir to a person.

Vaccine A preparation that stimulates an immune response that can prevent an infection or create resistance to an infection. Vaccines do not cause disease.

Vector A vector is a carrier of disease agents.

Viral infection The disease state resulting from the invasion of the body by a virus that can cause illness in humans.

Virus A particle composed of a piece of genetic material (RNA or DNA), surrounded by a protein coat. Viruses can reproduce only in living cells.

Waterborne bacterial disease An illness due to infection with bacteria from a contaminated water supply.

Widal test A tube agglutination test employed in the serological diagnosis of enteric fever.

Zoonoses An infectious disease that is transmissible from animals to humans under normal conditions.

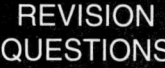

Revision Questions

CHAPTER 1
Concepts of Health and Disease

1. What do you mean by 'health'? Explain different concepts of health.
2. Explain the concepts of 'disease' and 'prevention of disease'.
3. Discuss the different models for health description.
4. Give a brief account of different determinants of health.
5. What do you mean by "Incidence Rate", "Prevalence Rate" and "Case fatality Rate".
6. Explain the 'primordial prevention'? How far is it important in prevention of disease?
7. How do the following differ:
   (a) Mental health and Spiritual health
   (b) Determinants of health and Indicators of health
   (c) Health and Disease
   (d) Pre-pathogenesis and Pathogenesis phases
8. Describe the role of heredity and environment as determinants of health.
9. Write short note on:
   (a) Physical health
   (b) Social health
   (c) Tertiary prevention
   (d) Holistic concept
10. What are indicators of health? Explain different indicators and their uses.
11. Explain the terms "Crude death rate", "Age and sex specific death rate" and "Infant mortality rate".

12. Explain the concept of disease and discuss the two phases in the natural history of disease.
13. Draw and explain the Iceberg of disease.
14. Critically examine the different definitions of health.
15. Classify the etiological factors and discuss their role in the occurrence of disease.
16. Give your views on 'Health Care in India – Vision 2020'.
17. Explain briefly:
    (a) Dynamic concept of health
    (b) Physical health
    (c) Life style as a determinant of health
    (d) Mental health
    (e) Natural history of health
    (f) Virulence
18. Write note on:
    (a) Concept of health
    (b) Sullivan's index
    (c) Primordial prevention
    (d) Mortality index
    (e) Holistic concept
    (f) Spiritual health
    (g) Concept of disease
    (h) Morbidity indicators.
    (i) Germ theory of disease.
19. Discuss the important concepts of health.
20. Give a brief account of models for health description.

CHAPTER 2

Nutrition and Health

1. Define the terms 'food' and 'nutrition' and explain their importance in 'health for all'.
2. Give a classification of foods.
3. Discuss briefly the nutritional requirements of adults.
4. What diseases are caused due to the deficiency of proteins? What is RDA of proteins?
5. How can protein-deficiency diseases be treated?
6. What measures should be taken to prevent protein-energy malnutrition?
7. Give a classification of vitamins.
8. Discuss the functions of vitamin A and describe the associated deficiency diseases.
9. Write a note on sources, daily requirements and over consumption of vitamin A.

10. Discuss the functions of vitamin D and describe the associated deficiency diseases.
11. Give the sources, daily requirement and over consumption of vitamin D.
12. Discuss the functions of vitamin E and describe the associated deficiency diseases.
13. Give the sources, daily requirement and over consumption of vitamin E.
14. Discuss the functions of vitamin K and describe the associated deficiency diseases.
15. Write about sources, daily requirement and over-consumption of vitamin K.
16. Discuss the functions of vitamin B_1 (thiamine) and describe the associated deficiency diseases.
17. Give the functions of niacin, sources, daily requirement and describe the associated deficiency diseases.
18. Describe the functions of vitamin B_6, sources, daily requirement and describe the associated deficiency diseases.
19. Describe the functions of folic acid, sources, daily requirement and describe the associated deficiency diseases.
20. Discuss the functions of vitamin C (ascorbic acid), sources, RDA and describe the associated deficiency diseases.
21. What are micronutrients and macronutrients?
22. What minerals are required by the body? Discuss their role in maintenance of health and give their recommended daily intake.
23. Describe the function, sources, daily requirement and the associated deficiency diseases of the following:
    (a) Calcium   (b) Magnesium
    (c) Phosphorus   (d) Sodium and potassium
    (e) Fluoride
24. Write about iodine and iron deficiency diseases.
25. Define balanced diet and give the balanced diet for adult male and female as recommended by ICMR.
26. Write note on:
    (a) Nutritional levels   (b) Nutritional requirements
    (c) Kwashiorkor   (d) Marasmus
    (e) Vitamin C   (f) PMN
    (g) Goitre   (h) Vitamin B complex
27. (a) Give three examples each of marketed products of Vitamin A, D, E and K.
    (b) Give three examples each of marketed products of vitamins B_1, B_2, B_5, B_6 and B_{12}.
    (c) Give five examples each of marketed products of different minerals, and multivitamins + minerals.
28. Explain the importance of pantothenic acid, ascorbic acid and folic acid in human health.
29. What is the role of biotin and niacin in human health?
30. Give a brief account of macrominerals and trace elements in human health.

CHAPTER 3
Demography and Family Planning

1. Define demography and give the demography of India.
2. Explain demographic cycle with its different stages.
3. Discuss various factors responsible for boosting the fertility rate in India.
4. How can high fertility rate in India be brought down?
5. What do you mean by family planning? Enumerate its various activities.
6. Discuss the objectives and scope of family planning in India.
7. What do you mean by "contraception", "contragestion", and "abortion"?
8. Compare the different types of contraception methods.
9. Discuss behavioural methods of contraception.
10. Discuss physical methods of contraception.
11. What is diaphragm? Discuss different types of diaphragm with their features.
12. Discuss chemical methods of contraception.
13. Briefly describe 'injectable contraceptives', and 'subdermal implants'.
14. Give a brief account of hormonal contraceptives.
15. Discuss the natural family planning methods.
16. Explain the permanent methods of contraception with suitable figures.
17. What do you mean by vasectomy and tubectomy? Discuss their role in birth control.
18. State the population problem of India and give your suggestions to solve it.
19. Write a note on census of India.
20. Write note on:
    (a) Nirodh   (b) IUDs
    (c) Copper T   (d) Rhythm method
    (e) Population equation   (f) Oral pills
    (g) Recommended family planning methods
21. Explain different stages of demographic cycle.
22. Briefly describe modern oral pills for contraception.
23. Briefly describe modern depot formulations for contraception.
24. What is the role of copper in contraception? Explain different types of copper devices.
25. Describe briefly the post-contraception methods.

CHAPTER 4
First-Aid

1. Define first-aid. Give a list of conditions when first-aid is required.
2. What are the objectives of a first-aid training programme?
3. What are the aims of first-aid?
4. What do you mean by ABCs of first-aid?

5. What is shock? Describe the symptoms and first-aid treatment of shock.
6. Explain the first-aid treatment of electric shock.
7. Recommend the emergency treatment in case of burn.
8. Suggest emergency treatment of poisoning.
9. Give comment on swallowed poisons and their first-aid.
10. Comment on inhalation poisoning and eye poisoning with their treatments.
11. What are resuscitation methods? Explain the back-pressure-arm-lift method.
12. Explain mouth-to-mouth breathing method and external heart compression method.
13. What do you mean by fracture? Describe different types of fractures.
14. Give a comparative account of simple fracture and compound fracture.
15. Describe general steps which should be followed in suspected fracture.
16. Recommend first-aid treatment in the case of following fractures:
    (a) Leg   (b) Spine
    (c) Upper arm
17. Recommend first-aid treatment in the case of following fractures:
    (a) Thigh   (b) Forearm and wrist
    (c) Collar bone
18. Recommend first-aid treatment in the case of following fractures:
    (a) Ribs   (b) Hips
    (c) Knee cap
19. What are different types of wounds? Describe first-aid treatment of wounds.
20. Explain differences in fracture and dislocation.
21. What are dressings? Classify them and discuss in detail.
22. Write note on:
    (a) Artificial respiration   (b) External heart compression
    (c) Dislocation   (d) Sprain
23. Write note on:
    (a) Back-pressure-arm-lift method
    (b) First-aid of burns   (c) Primary wound dressing
    (d) Snake bite.   (e) Rules of first aid
24. Give first-aid treatment of common heart diseases.
25. Compare utility of OASIS Ultra Tri-Layer Matrix and Aquacel Hydrofiber Dressing.

CHAPTER 5

Environment and Health

1. What is the role of sanitation in human health?
2. Define 'safe water' and 'potable water'.
3. Write about the sources of water.
4. Describe hydrological cycle.
5. Discuss different types of wells for supply of water.

6. What are different sources of impurities in water?
7. Describe various organic and inorganic impurities present in water.
8. What are the hazards of polluted water?
9. Describe different waterborne diseases along with their causative agents.
10. Briefly describe different methods of water purification.
11. With the help of a neat diagram explain the working of a slow sand filter.
12. With the help of a neat diagram explain the working of a rapid sand filter.
13. Give a comparative account of slow and rapid sand filters.
14. Describe the principle of Paterson's rapid filter.
15. Write a brief note on Horrock's test, Iodine test and Orthotoludine test.
16. What are different methods of domestic purification of water?
17. With the help of a neat diagram explain the working of any one domestic water filter.
18. What chemicals are used for water purification?
19. What is air pollution? What are the chief impurities present in the air?
20. What are different sources of air pollution?
21. What are the general indicators of air pollution?
22. What are the methods of prevention and control of air pollution?
23. What is ventilation? Describe the systems of ventilation.
24. What do you mean by noise pollution? What are the ill-effects of noise pollution?
25. Describe the measures for prevention and control of noise pollution.
26. What are the requirements of good lighting? What are the ill effects of bad lighting?
27. What are the sources of refuse? Describe the different methods of disposal of refuse.
28. Write about transmission of infection through faeces and role of sanitation barrier in transmission of various infections.
29. What are the different methods of excreta disposal?
30. Explain the construction and working of a bored hole latrine.
31. Explain the construction and working of RCA latrine.
32. Explain the construction and working of a septic tank.
33. Describe the essential components of a water carriage/sewerage system.
34. Write about the proper disposal of sewage.
35. Explain the construction and working of an activated sludge unit.
36. Write about the modern sewage treatment plant.
37. What is medical entomology? How do arthropods transmit diseases?
38. Give a classification of arthropods and describe the methods of control of arthropods.
39. Describe the different diseases caused by common arthropods.
40. How are diseases transmitted by mosquito, house fly, fleas and rodents?
41. Write different stages of life cycle of housefly. Explain the anti-fly measures.
42. Write different stages of life cycle of mosquito.
43. Write different types of lice infesting the humans.

44. Write short notes on:
    (a) Aqua privy
    (b) Sulabh Sauchalaya
    (c) Water closet system
45. Write short notes on:
    (d) Biological Oxygen Demand (BOD) of sewage
    (e) Biaeration process
    (f) Zoonotic infections
46. Write short notes on:
    (g) Horrock's test
    (h) Orthotoulidine test
    (i) Hazards of polluted air.
47. Write comment on:
    (a) Air disinfection
    (b) Chlorination
    (c) Indirect lighting
48. Write comment on:
    (d) Sanitation
    (e) Tube wells
    (f) Composting
    (g) Sanitation barrier
49. Write comment on:
    (h) Vital layer
    (i) Antirodent measures
    (j) Dug well latrine
    (k) Indicators of air pollution
    (l) Pasteur-Chamberland filter.
50. How can noise pollution in urban areas be minimized?

CHAPTER 6
Fundamental Principles of Microbiology

1. Give a brief history of microbiology.
2. Explain different systems of classification of bacteria.
3. Explain the similarity index.
4. Give classification of fungi.
5. Give causative organisms of the various disease: Candidiasis, Histoplasmosis, Aspergillosis, Ringworm, and Athlete's foot.
6. Write about the rickettsial diseases of human.
7. What are viruses? Enumerate their structure.
8. How can microorganisms be identified?
9. Describe the differences between eukaryotic and prokaryotic bacteria.
10. What are different forms of spherical/rod-shaped bacteria?

11. Explain the structure of a bacterial cell with the help of a neat labelled diagram.
12. What is the purpose of isolation of bacteria?
13. Explain the pure culture technique for isolation of bacteria.
14. Write a brief note on staining of bacteria.
15. Describe the advantages of staining of bacteria.
16. What are the different types of staining?
17. Explain the procedure of Ziehl-Neelsen staining.
18. Explain the procedure of traditional Gram staining.
19. What are the three steps in Gram staining?
20. What are the important differences between Gram (+)ve and Gram (–)ve bacteria?
21. Explain hanging drop method to observe live microorganisms.
22. Write the names of commonly used dyes for staining of microorganisms.
23. Write the steps of smear preparation.
24. Give the examples of Gram (+)ve and Gram (–)ve bacteria.
25. Write a note on medical applications of Gram staining.
26. Explain the acid-fast staining with its applications.
27. How Ziehl-Neelsen (Hot Stain) method differs from Kinyoun (Cold Stain) method?
28. What do you understand by negative staining? Give its procedural steps.
29. What is the endospore staining? Give its medical applications.
30. Explain the Graham & Evan's method of capsule staining.
31. Write about West and Difco's Spot test method. How it is useful in identifying bacterial species.

MULTIPLE CHOICE QUESTIONS (Right answers are underlined)

1. Rancidity in spoiled foods is due to:
   (a) <u>lipolytic organisms</u>.   (b) proteolytic organisms.
   (c) toxigenic microbes.   (d) saccharolytic microbes.
2. The bacterium most commonly used in genetic engineering is:
   (a) <u>*Escherichia*</u>.   (b) *Klebsiella*.
   (c) *Proteus*.   (d) *Serratia*.
3. The viruses that live as parasites on bacteria are called as:
   (a) fungi.   (b) commensals.
   (c) <u>bacteriophages</u>.   (d) None of these.
4. Gram positive bacteria can be stained by:
   (a) fast green.   (b) haematoxylin.
   (c) <u>crystal violet</u>.   (d) safranin.
5. Virus contains:
   (a) cell membrane.   (b) cell wall.
   (c) DNA.   (d) <u>DNA or RNA</u>.
6. Congenital diseases are:
   (a) <u>diseases present at birth</u>.   (b) deficiency diseases.
   (c) occur during life.
   (d) spread from one individual to another.

7. The site of energy production in a cell is:
  (a) micro body.
  (b) chromosome.
  (c) ribosome.
  (d) mitochondria.
8. Diphtheria is caused by:
  (a) *Corynebacterium.*
  (b) *Staphylococcus.*
  (c) *Streptococcus.*
  (d) None of these.
9. The most infectious food-borne disease is:
  (a) tetanus.
  (b) dysentery.
  (c) gas gangrene.
  (d) botulism.
10. An example of common air-borne epidemic disease is:
  (a) influenza.
  (b) typhoid.
  (c) encephalitis.
  (d) malaria.
11. Virion means:
  (a) infectious virus particles.
  (b) non-infectious particles.
  (c) incomplete particles.
  (d) defective virus particles.
12. The test used for detection of typhoid fever is:
  (a) Widal test.
  (b) ELISA.
  (c) Rosewaller test.
  (d) Western blotting.
13. The procedure of differential staining of bacteria was developed by:
  (a) Fleming.
  (b) Newton.
  (c) Gram.
  (d) Lister.
14. Gram staining is an example of:
  (a) simple staining.
  (b) differential staining.
  (c) negative staining.
  (d) None of these.
15. Rod-shaped bacteria are known as:
  (a) cocci.
  (b) comma forms.
  (c) bacilli.
  (d) pleomorphic forms.
16. The differences between Gram positive and Gram negative bacteria are shown to reside in the:
  (a) cell wall.
  (b) nucleus.
  (c) cell membrane.
  (d) mesosomes.
17. Bacteria multiply by:
  (a) spore formation.
  (h) binary fission
  (c) conjugation.
  (d) gametes.
18. The order of stains in Gram-staining procedure is:
  (a) crystal violet, iodine solution, alcohol, saffranine.
  (b) iodine solution, crystal violet, saffranine, alcohol.
  (c) alcohol, crystal violet, iodine solution, saffranine.
  (d) None of these.
19. Gram positive bacteria appear as:
  (a) pink.
  (b) violet.
  (c) Both a & b
  (d) None of these.
20. Gram negative bacteria appear as:
  (a) pink.
  (b) violet.
  (c) Both a & b.
  (d) None of these.

CHAPTER 7
Communicable Diseases

OBJECTIVE QUESTIONS (Right answers are bold)

1. A contagious disease is one that is mainly transmitted through:
   (a) vectors.   (b) fomites.
   (c) objects.   (d) **direct exposures.**
2. When a contagious disease suddenly increases in incidence it is said to be:
   (a) pandemic.   (b) **epidemic.**
   (c) endemic.   (d) sporadic.
3. A person who has direct association with an infected individual is classified as a:
   (a) susceptible.   (b) **contact.**
   (c) carrier.   (d) suspect
4. Contamination implies the presence of:
   (a) erythema.   (b) desquamation.
   (c) **pathogenic organism.**   (d) mosquitoes.
5. Pathognomonic means:
   (a) pathology of disease.
   (b) untoward symptoms.
   (c) prodromal signs.
   (d) **characteristic of a disease.**
6. An antigen is a substance which:
   (a) renders bacteria harmless.
   (b) neutralizes certain toxins.
   (c) produces local erythema.
   (d) **stimulates antibody production.**
7. The term enanthem refers to:
   (a) the toxin produced by a causative agent.
   (b) the systemic symptoms of a disease.
   (c) **the rash on the skin.**
   (d) the eruption on the mucosa.
8. A weakened toxin is called:
   (a) toxicide.   (b) **toxoid.**
   (c) toxicoid.   (d) toxicant.

TRUE OR FALSE (T – True; F – False)

1. Measles is transmitted by droplet infection.   **(T)**
2. Antiviral drugs are specifically used in the treatment of measles.   **(F)**
3. Tamiflu and Relenza are effective in influenza.   **(T)**
4. Trepenoma pallidum is the causative agent for syphilis.   **(T)**
5. Rabies is a zoonotic disease.   **(T)**

FILL IN THE BLANKS   (Right answers)

1. TB is a .... disease.   (bacterial)
2. Influenza is a .... disease.   (viral)
3. Cholera is a .... disease.   (bacterial)
4. Chickenpox is a .... disease.   (viral)
5. Leprosy is a .... disease.   (bacterial)
6. Malaria is a .... disease.   (protozoal)
7. Rabies is a .... disease.   (viral)
8. Tetanus is a .... disease.   (bacterial)
9. Measles is a .... disease.   (viral)
10. Trachoma is a .... disease.   (bacterial)

EXPAND THE FOLLOWING ABBREVIATIONS

1. DPT **(Diphtheria, Pertusis, Tetanus)**
2. EPI **(Expanded Program on Immunization)**
3. ORS **(Oral rehydration salts)**
4. WHO **(World Health Organization)**
5. ARV **(Anti-rabies vaccine)**
6. BPL **(β-Propiolactone)**
7. RDRV **(Rhesus cell strain rabies vaccine)**
8. NLCP **(The National Leprosy Control Program)**
9. STD **(Sexually transmitted disease)**
10. AIDS **(Acquired immune deficiency syndrome)**
11. HIV **(Human Immunodeficiency Virus)**
12. ELISA **(Enzyme-linked immunosorbent assay)**
13. RIA **(Radioimmunoassay)**
14. HAART **(Highly active antiretroviral therapy)**
15. ATS **(Anti-tetanus serum)**

DESCRIPTIVE QUESTIONS

EACH OF 1 MARK

1. Infective agent of chickenpox.
2. Infective agent of plague.
3. Infective agent of trachoma.
4. Infective agent of rabies.
5. Infective agent of AIDS.
6. Infective agent of diarrhoea.
7. Infective agent of pertusis.

EACH OF 2 MARKS

8. What are examples of bacterial infections?
9. Name five viral diseases.
10. Classification of communicable diseases.
11. Mode of transmission of chickenpox.

12. Mode of transmission of plague.
13. Mode of transmission of trachoma.
14. Mode of transmission of rabies.
15. Mode of transmission of AIDS.
16. Mode of transmission of diarrhoea.
17. Mode of transmission of pertusis.
18. What are common protozoal infections?
19. Describe immunization for measles.
20. Control and prevention of tetanus.
21. Vaccines for tuberculosis.

EACH OF 3 MARKS

22. What causes infections?
23. Signs and symptoms of measles.
24. What are common viral infections?
25. How are viral infections spread?
26. Signs and symptoms of polio.
27. Signs and symptoms of chickenpox.
28. Preventive measures for measles.
29. Preventive measures for polio.
30. Preventive measures for chickenpox.
31. Control measures for cholera.
32. Control measures for typhoid.
33. Control measures for dysentery.
34. Incubation and communicability of cholera.
35. Incubation and communicability of typhoid.
36. Incubation and communicability of dysentery.
37. Infective agent and preventive measures for TB.
38. Infective agent and preventive measures for pertusis.
39. Infective agent and preventive measures for tetanus.

EACH OF 5 MARKS

40. Describe 'chain of infection'.
41. Give the causative agents of communicable diseases with examples.
42. Describe different 'modes of transmission' of diseases.
43. Give the general principles for control of communicable diseases.
44. Mode of transmission and control measures for chickenpox.
45. Mode of transmission and control measures for diarrhoea.
46. Mode of transmission and control measures for tetanus.
47. Mode of transmission and control measures for malaria.
48. Mode of transmission and control measures for hookworm.
49. What is the host parasite environment relationship in transmission of communicable diseases?
50. Write short note on pertusis and tetanus.

CHAPTER 8
Non-communicable Diseases

MULTIPLE CHOICE QUESTIONS (Right answers are bold)

1. Normal vision is reported by:
   (a) 1/6. (b) **6/6.**
   (c) 6/1. (d) None.
2. Blindness is a state when a person is unable to count fingers in daylight at a distance of:
   (a) 6 metres. (b) 1 metre.
   (c) **3 metres.** (d) None.
3. Preferred for the care of acute attack of asthma:
   (a) Long-acting β-agonist. (b) **Bronchodilators.**
   (c) Both a and b. (d) None.
4. Stroke is diagnosed by:
   (a) MRI scans. (b) arteriography.
   (c) Doppler ultrasound. (d) **All.**
5. Biomarker used to diagnose the risk of cardiovascular disease:
   (a) Elevated blood levels of asymmetric dimethylarginine.
   (b) Higher fibrinogen.
   (c) Elevated homocysteine.
   (d) **All.**

TRUE OR FALSE (T – True; F – False)

6. In Type 1 diabetes body makes little or no insulin. **(T)**
7. Chemotherapy is not used with surgery in treatment of cancer. **(F)**
8. Type II diabetes is the most common form of diabetes mellitus. **(T)**
9. Diabetes insipidus and diabetes mellitus are hormonal disorders. **(T)**
10. Diabetes mellitus is a risk factor for chronic kidney diseases. **(T)**

FILL IN THE BLANKS

11. The characteristics of non-communicable diseases are .... and ....
    disease. **(long duration; slow progression)**
12. Diabetes is characterized by .... and ....
    (hyperglycemia; glycosuria)
13. Blindness can be defined as a state when vision becomes less than ....
    of normal vision. **(3/60ᵗʰ)**
14. A patient is likely to suffer with diabetes if his fasting blood glucose level
    is > .... mg/dL. **(126)**
15. Adequate intake of vitamin .... rich food helps in persistence of healthy
    eyes. **(A)**

EXPAND THE FOLLOWING ABBREVIATIONS FOR IMAGING METHODS

16. MRI **(Magnetic resonance imaging)**
17. CT **(Computed tomography)**
18. MAG3 **(Mercapto acetyl tri glycine)**
19. DMSA **(Technetium dimercaptosuccinic acid)**
20. SPECT **(Single photon emission tomography)**
21. PET **(Positron emission tomography)**

DESCRIPTIVE QUESTIONS

EACH OF 1 MARK

1. Define non-communicable diseases.
2. What is silent stroke?
3. Define blindness.
4. Give types of diabetes.
5. Define asthma.
6. What is Alzheimer's disease?

EACH OF 2 MARKS

7. Name the methods for diagnosis of asthma.
8. Name any four non-communicable diseases.
9. Give a list of diagnostic methods for strokes.
10. Differentiate between benign and malignant tumours.
11. Name the Regional Cancer Centres for prevention and control of cancer in India.
12. Write five risk factors for cardiovascular diseases.
13. Which methods are used for diagnosis of kidney diseases?
14. Differentiate between early onset and late onset of Alzheimer's disease.

EACH OF 3 MARKS

15. Describe treatment strategy for asthma.
16. Name the types of cardiovascular problems.
17. Define cancer and describe the causes of cancer.
18. Define diabetes and explain its etiology.
19. Discuss the symptoms of diabetes.
20. Describe the causes of blindness.
21. Give the prevention and control measures for cardiovascular problems.
22. Differentiate between ischemic stroke and hemorrhagic stroke.
23. Describe the treatment strategies for strokes.
24. Give the diagnosis method and prevention strategy for Alzheimer's disease.

EACH OF 5 MARKS

25. Classify kidney diseases giving the criteria for confirming that a patient is suffering from kidney diseases.

26. Give the pathophysiology risk factors, symptoms and treatment of Alzheimer's disease.
27. Discuss symptoms, diagnosis and treatment of cancer.
28. Discuss the diagnosis of cardiovascular diseases. Give a brief summary on the control and measures to prevent cardiovascular problems.
29. Discuss the diagnosis and treatment of diabetes mellitus.
30. Define 'stroke' and discuss its etiology, symptoms and risk factors.

CHAPTER 9
Epidemiology

MULTIPLE CHOICE QUESTIONS (Right answers are bold)

1. In epidemiological studies, pharmacists are concerned with:
   (a) communicable disease.   (b) non-communicable diseases.
   (c) **Both a and b.**   (d) None.
2. The intersection of host, agent and environment for analysis of an outbreak is termed as:
   (a) causal inference.   (b) **epidemiologic triad.**
   (c) biostatistics.   (d) biomonitoring.
3. An antiseptic is an agent that .... the growth of microorganisms.
   (a) supports   (b) inhibits
   (c) destroys   (d) **b and c**
4. Membrane filters with pore sizes between .... μm are commonly used to remove particles from solutions that can't be autoclaved.
   (a) **0.2–0.45**   (b) 200–450
   (c) 2000–4500   (d) None
5. As a method of disinfection, filtration .... the microbes.
   (a) supports   (b) inhibits
   (c) **removes**   (d) a and b

TRUE OR FALSE (T – True; F – False)

1. Berkefeld filters are made of Kieselguhr.   **(T)**
2. 40% formaldehyde (formalin) is used to disinfect wool.   **(F)**
3. Triclosan has good activity against Gram positive bacteria.   **(T)**
4. Antigen could be anything that can trigger the immune response.   **(T)**
5. Monocytes are phagocytes that circulate in the blood.   **(T)**

FILL IN THE BLANKS

1. The main objectives of epidemiology are ...., ... and complete .... of disease from human race. **(prevention, control, eradication)**
2. Study of cause of the disease is called .... **(etiology)**

3. Communicable diseases are transmitted from .... of infection to the .... by different modes of transmission.
   (source/reservoir, susceptible host)
4. Disinfection is a less lethal process than .... **(sterilization)**
5. A disinfectant in .... concentration can be used as antiseptic. **(low)**

EXPAND THE FOLLOWING ABBREVIATIONS FOR IMAGING METHODS

1. AIDS **(Acquired immuno deficiency syndrome)**
2. STDs **(Sexually transmitted diseases)**
3. CDCs **(Centers for Disease Control and Prevention)**
4. WHO **(World Health Organization)**
5. DOP **(Dioctylphthalate)**
6. HEPA **(High Efficiency Particle Air filters)**
7. BPL **(Beta-Propiolactone)**
8. RW **(Rideal-Walker coefficient)**
9. NK cells **(Natural killer cells)**
10. MHC **(Major histocompatibility complex)**
11. TCR **(T cell receptor)**
12. APCs **(Antigen-presenting cells)**

DESCRIPTIVE QUESTIONS

EACH OF 1 MARK

1. Classify the study designs in epidemiology.
2. Describe the salient features of epidemiology.
3. Define 'descriptive epidemiology'.
4. What is 'experimental epidemiology'?
5. Define the terms 'infection' and 'disease'.
6. What are communicable diseases?
7. Describe the types of autoclave?
8. What is antigen?

EACH OF 2 MARKS

1. Define epidemiology. Discuss its objectives and aims.
2. Name some of the normal flora present in the skin and large intestine of human body.
3. What is pathology?
4. Describe analytical epidemiology.
5. Enlist the components and steps in the epidemiology.
6. Discuss the areas included in epidemiology in the disease of study.
7. Discuss the components (pre-requisites) of disease transmission.
8. Enlist the events involved in disease transmission.
9. Discuss the Koch's hypothesis or discuss the etiology of infectious diseases.
10. Differentiate between vertical and horizontal modes of transmission.

11. Enlist the strategies for controlling a disease.
12. Give the mechanisms by which disinfectants works.
13. What is cold sterilization?

EACH OF 3 MARKS

14. Discuss about the Bradford-Hill criteria.
15. Discuss "causal inference".
16. Compare cohort studies with case control studies.
17. Give a brief report on population-based health management.
18. Discuss in brief about the normal flora and host relationship and opportunistic infections.
19. Give a brief report on the steps involved in the development of disease.
20. Compare direct and indirect transmission.
21. What do you mean by isolation period? Give the recommended isolation period for some communicable diseases.
22. Give a report on the measures recommended by CDC and WHO to prevent emerging infectious diseases.
23. What are portals of exit for microbes?
24. What are nosocomial infections?
25. Describe the types of infections.
26. Enlist the factors affecting sterilization by heat.
27. Differentiate between ionizing and non-ionizing rays for radiation sterilization.
28. Write a note on HEPA filters.
29. Classify chemical disinfectants.
30. Discuss the mechanism of action and applications of halogens as disinfectants.
31. Differentiate between Rideal-Walker test and Chick-Martin test.
32. Compare the Kelsey-Sykes test with Rideal-Walker test.
33. Discuss the utility of "in-use dilution" test for disinfection testing.
34. What is immunity? How do immune systems differentiate between "self" and "non-self" components?
35. Discuss the different layers of protection.
36. Differential between T cells and B cells as components of immune systems.
37. Differential between innate and adaptive immune systems.
38. Differential between helper T cells and cytotoxic T cells.
39. What is immune tolerance?
40. Discuss various disorders of immune system with special emphasis on autoimmune diseases.

EACH OF 5 MARKS

41. Discuss the study designs and methods of epidemiology.
42. Differentiate between case series and case control studies.

43. Differentiate between prospective study (cohort study) and retrospective study (case control study).
44. Discuss the uses of epidemiological studies in health system.
45. What are emerging infectious diseases? Name any seven emerging infectious diseases with their causative microorganisms.
46. Classify the infectious diseases on different basis.
47. What are reservoirs of infection? What do you mean by carrier in a communicable disease?
48. Describe the chain of infection as well as the means of breaking this chain to prevent infection.
49. What are different modes of transmission of communicable diseases?
50. Give a report on the measures to control communicable diseases.
51. Discuss the factors involved in the spread of Nosocomial infections. Give a note on the measures to prevent these infections.
52. Write a note on methods of disinfection.
53. What is moist heat sterilization? Give the principle, mechanism and working of an autoclave.
54. Discuss the different types of filters.
55. Mention the properties of ideal disinfectants.
56. Compare aldehydes and phenols as disinfectants.
57. Give the methods for testing disinfectants with special emphasis on Rideal-Walker method.
58. Give a report on the components of immune system.
59. What is phagocytosis? Discuss the role of different cells in this process.
60. What is the source of antibodies? Discuss their types and functions.
61. What is immunity? Differentiate between natural and acquired immunity.
62. Write a note on immunization with description of national immunization schedule and expanded program of immunization.
63. Describe the disinfection procedures for:
    (a) Faeces and urine
    (b) Sputum
    (c) Room
64. How do the following differ?
    (a) Sterilization and disinfection
    (b) Antigen and antibody
    (c) Active and passive immunity
65. Describe the disinfection procedures for:
    (a) Linen
    (b) Instruments
    (c) Dead bodies

INDEX

Index